Practice Positive

**A Simple Guide to Becoming a
Positive and Happy Person**

By Dawn Carson

Dear Adam
may all good things
come to you and only
good things come to
you. And it will
be true if your
eyes stay open

love Dan

Practice Positive
Copyright © 2013 Dawn Carson

Library and Archives Canada Cataloguing in Publication

Carson, Dawn, 1976-, author
        Practice positive : a simple guide to becoming a positive
and happy person / Dawn Carson.

ISBN 978-0-9919546-0-5 (pbk.)

        1. Happiness. 2. Well-being. 3. Depression,
Mental Health--
Popular works. I. Title.

    BF575.H27C37 2013   158   C2013-
903147-2

Bliss Bomb Publishing
17273 58 Avenue
  ʼrrey, BC V3S 1K7

    ʼ in Canada

Testimonials

"This book comes to me in a form of pure honesty and kind sharing. The writer has gone through many challenges in life and has found ways to get through them that are holistic and positive. I am "Grateful" to have read this book and see that no matter what circumstances happen in your life that there are ways to overcome and rise above – we are in control of our life and Dawn Carson has shared how we can make our life better and happier. This book is inspiring from beginning to end and I know that if she can do it then so can I and so can you."

-Trina Goebel
Owner, That Spa & Nail Place

"A very insightful and inspiring piece on the powers of positive thinking. The author's message is clear and one we should all take stock: If we can learn to think more positive (even when things don't always go our way) then our lives and personal experiences will reflect this. Sometimes in the hustle and bustle of life we forget to stop and reflect even in the smallest joys in life, but the author reminds us even the smallest joys will add up and bring happiness."

-Jason Trenchard
Owner/Operator, Allpro Landscaping

Dedication

To the four most important ladies in my life:

Myrtle Carson – my grandma. For her constant encouragement.

Raejoan Slusarenko – my mom. For being my rock in the darkest of times, and my friend all the rest of the time.

Lynda Carson – my second mom. For teaching me that there is beauty in the details.

Angelina Carson – my niece. For reminding me to embrace my inner child and have fun, just because I can.

Disclaimer

Table of Contents

Foreword

"By leaving your comfort zone behind and taking a leap of faith into something new, you find out who you are truly capable of becoming."

- Unknown

Dawn Carson's <u>Practice Positive:</u> *a simple guide to becoming a positive and happy person,* is exactly that – a simple, clear and effective guide to help you find ways to be more positive and to live a happier life.

Like many, Dawn's life journey has taken her through major life shifts. Since she and I met a few years ago in a wellness center, where we worked, I have observed her grow from someone who was working through depression; low self-confidence, frozen and unable to move or make a decision; into a woman who is learning to take action when she recognizes the signs that used to bring her down. A woman who asks for help, and gets out there and finds what shifts her vibration up because she knows what she has to do and that she's the only one who can do the work. Allowing the confidence to come out from within her – for it was always there. She just had to discover it. Learning how to be more positive was key in leading Dawn into herself.

There are many wonderful self-help books. So how do you decide where to begin? Dawn's philosophy? Just start. In <u>Practice Positive</u>, she shares her own experiences on how to find the positive in your life and why it's important to do so. It is packed full of practical ideas, that meet a variety of interests, needs, and budgets. This informative and easy to read guide takes the mystery out of what to do when you are feeling negative, stuck in a rut and just can't seem to get yourself to try something new to you. Some step by step suggestions such as: downsizing negativity in your life, how to add in easy and manageable positive actions, how to be grateful, how to discover hobbies, interests, movement and music, and various other creative techniques that feed and nurture your soul.

Dawn reminds you to take small steps, assess where you are, and be realistic and honest with yourself. From surrounding yourself with support to trying something new, you can't do it wrong. Just take action and try something. If you don't like it, then stop doing it and choose another. And it is about choice, as well as practice and patience. You get to choose what you like to do, and then do it.

Take a risk and allow yourself to learn to play again and to unveil things about yourself that you may not even know exist. Embrace who you are – you are worth the changes you are making! Let <u>Practice Positive</u> be a key to helping you discover many ways to enhance and bring more joy into your life.

With Love and Gratitude

Virginia Smith BGS, RT-CRA
Reiki Master/Teacher/Practitioner
Vice-President, Canadian Reiki Association

Preface

In late 2006 I experienced a breakdown of my mental health. I fell into a deep depression. I was filled with anxiety and dark thoughts. I checked myself into psychiatric care at the local hospital for my safety, as I had become suicidal.

I learned many things during my six week stay in the psych ward. Unfortunately I left the facility on a large amount of medications and was virtually a zombie. I was unable to function in society that way, so over the course of a year I weaned myself off all the prescription drugs.

I felt better physically but my mind was still plagued with anxiety and depression. I researched many alternative remedies and therapies to battle these troubled feelings. I read a variety of books and articles to find methods that worked for me.

This book is the result of over four years of personal research. I decided to share what I have learned because, had I found one book that had all of this information in it, my recovery would have been much faster. I hope that this book aids you in your path to happiness.

Introduction

The main goal of this book is to present you with ways to become happier. Where you are at in your life now will effect how quickly you are able to approach and embrace happiness and positivity. Be patient with yourself. If you are in the depths of depression I salute you for even picking up this book in the first place.

If you are feeling very low right now then use this book to slowly improve your mood. Think of the things I suggest as ways to raise your positivity in small increments. I like to call this *Leveling Up*. On a scale of 1 to 5 rate how you feel. A 1 represents the lowest of the low. If you are at level 1 then don't shoot for being a level 5 right away. That will only make you feel hopelessly discouraged. Instead, aim for a 1.5 or a 2. Slow and steady is the pace to set.

Sadness is a low feeling. If you are sad right now, work on improving that feeling by just a little bit. Feel the best you can at this moment. Continue to work on doing that and eventually things will improve. Also, if you 'backslide' give yourself a break. It isn't failure to go backwards. Sometimes your body and mind just need to take a step back in order to process what you have been doing. There is no shame in that.

We are all on our own path. Make sure you allow yourself to progress the way you are meant to. There is no need to rush. There is no need to compare yourself to others. You don't even need to compare yourself with who you once were. Who you are now is the most important thing to embrace. You can improve and grow as much as you want to. It just takes patience and a little self-love.

Use this book as a guide or resource. Find the things in it that work for you right now. Other things may work later on. Just make small changes and embrace the journey. Trust that your body and mind will allow the changes to take hold when you are truly ready. Above all have as much fun as you can.

The world is full of a lot of fear, and a lot of negativity, and a lot of judgment. I just think people need to start shifting into joy and happiness. As corny as it sounds, we need to make a shift.

- Ellen Degeneres

Chapter 1

Erasing Negativity

In order to embrace positivity in your life, it is essential that you first erase or limit negativity from it. You can't fill up an already full tank. You need to create space for the new. There are many ways to do this. I suggest making a list of areas in your life that are the most negative and start from there. Take some time to write out the things you deal with regularly that are negative. Rank them from 1 to 5 on a scale of negativity and then choose an area to start working on. It doesn't matter how high the area ranks. This just tells you the areas that are the biggest problem for you. You don't need to start working on the mountain. You can start with a molehill.

Little Details Matter

It is important to look at the small things we do as much as the big things. Small things can add up to Big Negativity, which of course is what we are working to avoid. Things like our choice in music and TV shows can greatly effect our emotions. Music is an area that can be pretty sneaky at being negative. Sometimes the background music itself will sound very upbeat, but the words may be really awful. The reverse can be true as well. Some of the darkest sounding music can have a neutral or even positive message.

Words are very important so if the music you listen to the most has really negative lyrics, I suggest you take a break from it or stop listening to it entirely. Yes this can be frustrating, but your emotional world is affected powerfully by words. As for the darker sounding music that has a neutral or positive message, you may need to keep track of a few things to figure out if you need to toss this stuff. Keep a journal on music for a week or two. Write how you feel before the music is put on, while you listen and afterwards. If you are feeling low every time you choose this particular music, and don't feel any better after listening to it, toss it. It is just reinforcing your low mood. If you feel better in any way from listening to it then it's probably fine.

With the huge variety of music available I'm sure you can find something positive and uplifting to listen to. If you are finding this task a bit too daunting, work on a different area of your life first. Music is a very personal thing for some people, so you may need to raise your positive vibration a bit all round before you decide to chuck your CD collection.

TV and movies are another big area that negativity can easily creep into. If you are prone to watching violent and dark shows, or shows that increase your level of stress while watching them, you may need to rethink what you watch. Find shows with humour and a lighter message in them. There are a lot of great shows out there that aren't particularly violent or negative. I'm not saying you can't ever watch your favourite shows again, just find some balance. Again, you can always use the journaling technique to gage whether this is an area you need to clean up or not. If you regularly feel crappy or tense during or after watching your shows then I do suggest you stop watching them.

You don't necessarily need to give up war movies and horror shows completely. It really is more about balance than a clean sweep. Small changes all add up to better things. Make the majority of what you listen to and watch positive, humorous and intelligent. Think of it as a set of scales. On one side are the negative things we do and on the other side are the positive things that benefit us. You just need to be doing enough to increase your positivity, to shift those scales so that the positive side is greater than the negative side most of the time.

One thing that I strongly suggest you stop watching is the news. Stop reading newspapers too. This advice may surprise you as people really feel that it is important to keep in the loop of what is going on in the world. But here's the thing, they are filled with about as much negativity as you can find anywhere in a single place. If you really think about it you can probably predict what is going on anyways: someone got shot, there's been another teen shooting, there is a war overseas, bombs are going off...you get the idea. The actual stories may be different but the content is still the same. And it is all pretty much negative. Plus, you can't do a whole lot to change any of it yourself, so why do you need to know all of this stuff every day? This may seem like a really big thing to give up but the benefits will definitely outweigh the loss.

Trust me. I haven't watched the news regularly in 15 years. It is probably the best decision I have ever made for my well-being. I tune in from time to time to watch a political debate or find out more on a topic I heard about from someone at work (i.e.: 9-11) but for the most part I avoid it. I still find myself 'in the loop', as anything I really need to know about I hear from friends and family members. I also encounter quite a bit of news through social media and perfect strangers in grocery lineups! You will too.

There are exceptions to this 'rule'. Local community newspapers are often valuable resources of information on what is going on in your town. They tend to run articles on local events and people. This fosters a great sense of community and can help you feel connected. The other exception is the entertainment and sports pages of larger newspapers. Their main focus is on fun things to do. This is obviously a wonderful way to find events in your area to raise your positivity, as well as new music, books and the like.

Gossip

Ok this is an uncomfortable topic to broach. Gossip. No one really likes to say they engage in it, but the majority of people do. At least from time to time. We talk smack about our coworkers, friends, hookups, drinking debacles, celebrities, politicians and everything in between. Everyone loves a scandal.

Gossip can be a way for people to bond. It serves its purpose I suppose, in bringing people together against a common denominator. Seriously though? I think we can probably find better use of our time and energy. Why not put our heads together and come up with creative solutions to the worlds problems? Too heavy? Then find something positive to talk about, like your hobby, your cat, the last movie you saw, a class you are taking...you get the idea.

The fact is that the more time we spend speaking about nasty, negative things (GOSSIP) the more negativity we are spreading in our own lives and the lives of others. No one wins. Negativity breeds negativity. Period. So do what you can to limit the amount of time you are immersing yourself in gossip. Now I'm not saying you can't talk about the hot guy in your tech department at work, or the babe at the bakery. If there is a positive spin on it (i.e. talent, sexiness) go for it. That isn't negative, that's spreading some pretty nice information. Nothing really wrong with that. Just leave the biting, jealous, cruel comments where they belong. Nowhere.

This may be difficult at first. Gossip, like so many things we do, is a habit and can take some effort to break free from. Be patient with yourself. Don't beat yourself up every time you slip up here. That isn't going to raise your level of positivity. Instead see it as a process. Take it day by day and eventually you'll find that it becomes less of a habit and more of an occasional activity. If you find yourself inundated with gossip from friends, coworkers or family members, tell them you really want to curb the habit. Lots of people will be supportive of your efforts to better yourself. They may even want to do it with you. If you do find that some people will simply not quit, divert the conversations to a new topic, or just walk away if you have to. It will suck at first but people will learn to respect your desire to be more positive. It just may take some time. Change is never an immediate thing. Stick to it and things will improve. You and everyone around you will benefit in the end.

Self-Talk

One area that many people struggle with negativity in is Self-Talk. We are our own worst critics. We look at ourselves in the mirror and think all sorts of awful things about ourselves. We hate our thighs, our skinny arms, our less than perfect abs. We have bad hair, dull skin and crooked teeth. There are probably things that everyone can find to complain about themselves. This is an area that is common and destructive. Let's work on changing that.

The thoughts and words we use to describe ourselves are powerful. If you are regularly putting yourself down, it is time to stop. You need to start looking at yourself as more than just a body. That is far too simplistic a view. You are a mind, a creative force, a miracle of science, a spirit. You have so much to offer this world. Through your unique ideas, interests and passions you help shape this world into a very cool place.

You may not be aware of what your talents are, what others admire and like about you, what you add to the world. Here's a novel idea.

Ask people. Send out an email or a Facebook post asking people to tell you the quality they like most about you. You will probably be surprised by the variety of comments you receive. This is a really great way to help you see how *others* see you, instead of just focusing on how *you* see you. We tend to focus only on the parts of ourselves that we don't like. Our friends and family often focus more heavily on what they love about us. How's that for finding a balanced and accurate view of ourselves!

Your body is pretty amazing too. Who cares if you don't look like a model on the cover of a magazine? Newsflash! They don't look like that either. Airbrushing and a tonne of makeup is what you are seeing on those pages. It's really just a giant lie. As for celebrities, comparing yourself to a person who has the income to pay for personal chefs and trainers to keep them on track is ridiculous. It's their JOB to look amazing. I'm guessing your job is slightly different than that. You probably get paid to do something a bit more important than looking good. I'm just saying!

There is a slightly brutal technique you can use to help you kick the habit of negative self-talk. It is a technique that requires *specialist equipment*. It takes an Elastic Band. Put a thick elastic band on your wrist. A thick one works best because it needs to hurt when you snap it.

There are two ways to do this. The first is to simply snap the elastic band every time you catch yourself saying, or thinking something mean or demeaning about yourself. Your brain will begin to equate pain with negative self-talk and you will eventually stop talking smack like that. The second way starts the same, but after you snap the elastic band, state something great about yourself. No hesitation. This will not only equate pain with negativity, but it will also reprogram your brain to use positive self-talk. It serves to shock the mind, then install a positive thought in place of the negative one. This is a really effective technique. The more often you do this the faster you will *believe* the positive statements you are saying. If you have trouble thinking of positive things about yourself on the fly, make a list of go-to statements that you can memorize, or recall the things your friends and family members said about you. Here are some examples of how this will go with the second method.

"I am so stupid" SNAP "I am an intelligent person".

"My thighs are fat" SNAP "I am beautiful".

"I can't ever do anything right" SNAP "I am completely capable".

Remember, the snap has to hurt. Thwack that rubber band like your life depends on it. Actually it kind of does! Your level of positivity needs to increase in order for your life to be better and for you to be happier.

Words of Caution

Self-talk can be a really big problem. Something you may not realize is that certain words are also a big problem in the form of self-talk. Words such as 'try', 'can't', 'should' and 'hate' can be devastating to your psyche. Let's start with the word *try*. Oh how this word gets us into trouble.

Try

When we say 'I'm trying to eat healthier" or "I'll try to get the project done on time" what we are actually doing is pretty complex, and ultimately negative. You see, in these cases, *TRY* implies doubt. It puts a seed of doubt right in your mind, stating that the very thing you want to do, may not be possible to do. The only reason to use the word try, which is positive, is when you are talking about trying something new. 'I'm trying Vietnamese food for the first time today.' 'I'm going to try golf this weekend.'

These are statements that are simply fact, and have no doubt attached to them. See the difference? Avoid 'trying' to do anything that is not new and exciting. Instead, own what you are doing and say things like "I'm working at making healthy eating a habit" and "I plan to have the project done on time". These statements put you in a position of power and are far more positive. It's actually better to tell someone that you will *not* do something than to say you will try to, and then not do it.

Can't

This is a contraction that needs to be abolished from the English language unless used correctly. Can't is meant to be used to convey factual impossibility as in "I can't see" or "I can't hear" or 'I can't go (as in I'm not allowed). Unfortunately we use it in conversation to state fear or unwillingness. It implies you have no choice in the matter. This is just crap. Plain and simple. You always have a choice in your behaviour. Period. Sure the choice may be painful or embarrassing but it is still a choice.

Saying you can't succeed, can't lose weight, can't make friends, can't get a job is a copout. You may not know *how* you will do these things. You may not have any experience in these things. You may not even *want* to do these things. Regardless, you can and are choosing not to. Really you are just saying" I Won't". So own it. Be honest with yourself about what limitations are in your head, what fears you have and move on. You Can.

Should

This is another tough one. Should generally implies guilt. This does nothing to improve your positivity. If you feel guilty, that's bad. The proper way to use the word should is when asking a question as in "Should I do step 3 before step 4 in the experiment?" or "Should I bring anything to the party?" We tend to use the word should in an entirely different manner. We say things like "I should exercise" and "We should probably go" and "I shouldn't eat that". This is a problem because it implies that you are bad if you don't exercise. It implies that you don't want to go but feel you have to. It implies that you are naughty if you eat what you are wanting to.

Do you see how this word can be toxic to you? It takes away all of your power! Why not say instead "I need to exercise" and "I'm going to go because I'm getting up early tomorrow" and "I'm not going to eat that because I'm committed to getting healthier". Own what you do. Not out of guilt, but out of your own self-worth; your pride. That is a much more positive way of dealing with things.

Hate

Certain words hold a lot more energy than others. Hate is one of those words. Hate is a very strong emotion. When you use the word hate in conversation, even in a flippant way, you are playing with fire. Be mindful of how often you use this word. If it is something you say on a regular basis you may just end up getting burned.

It has become common practice for people to throw words like love and hate around like they aren't as powerful as they actually are. Unfortunately these words *are* powerful. They hold so much emotional attachment to them that when we use them casually we are in danger of misunderstanding just how potent they can be.

Every word you say originates in your thoughts. When you are in the habit of using words like loathing, despising and hating, that means that your thoughts are on those things way too often. Your thought-life creates your physical life. We get what we focus on the most. If you are focusing on how much you dislike or hate something, then you will find more things to hate. It's that simple.

This is why I included gratitude as a whole chapter in this book! If you instead focus on things that you love and are grateful for, more of those things will show up in your life. So what do you want? Focus on those things to raise your positivity. Chuck out the words should, try, can't and hate and see how much happier you become.

Emotional Vampires

If you find that when you spend time with friends the chatter is filled with complaining, gossip and the like, it may be a good time to start cleaning house. This can mean simply not engaging in negative talk or changing the subject perhaps. It may mean spending less time with these friends and finding new friends who are more positive. This may be necessary to find balance. It may even mean cutting out certain friends from your life entirely. I understand that this can be a really hard choice. I've had to do it myself a few times. You need to look at the big picture and decide if overall this friendship nourishes and uplifts you, or if it deteriorates you.

Some people are what I like to call Emotional Vampires. They suck all the good out of life. And that is not good. These people are not your run-of-the-mill friends who are just in a tough spot right now. These people are chronically negative. It is like they are just unhappy to the core. No amount of encouragement changes their attitude. They just aren't at a healthy place in life and they only bring you down.

If you have friends like this you need to seriously evaluate whether this friendship is something you can continue, and still increase your positivity. If this is a family member, you'll probably need to limit your time with them. It may be necessary to only spend time with these people in a group. Regardless of how you choose to handle them, do not engage in their negativity. I also suggest you give up on the idea that you can change them. It is a daunting task that most likely will only end with you feeling low, drained and emotionally exhausted. Not worth it. They will change when they are ready to, if ever. Remember, it is only your job to take care of *you*. That is everyone else's job too.

It is a really good idea to develop a support system or network of people who are generally positive and uplifting. Spend quality time with family members who are encouraging and inspiring. Find new friends who are upbeat and choose to be happy most of the time. Everyone has ups and downs, but if the overall mood of a person is positive, then they are the perfect kind of person to spend lots of time with. Your personal outlook on life is directly affected by the people you spend the majority of your time with. If you are spending time laughing a tonne, you are with the right people. If you leave friends and family and find yourself smiling on the way home, you are with the right people. It's actually pretty simple. Cling to those people who raise your positivity. Stick to them like glue.

A Note On Complaining

If you are prone to frequent bouts of complaining I urge you to stop. Every time you complain about something or someone you are putting a lot of negative energy behind your words. All this leads to are more things to complain about. Your emotions will be predominantly negative and it will only lead to more problems. Besides, no one really wants to hear you complain anyways. It is both boring and irritating to the listener when all you have to add to conversation are complaints. If you make it a habit to leave your complaints to yourself, perhaps others will as well.

Slow and Steady

Keep in mind that you do not need to make all of these changes at once. Take time to get used to one small change before moving onto the next one. This will help ensure your success, and make the transition much smoother and less painful. Change can be overwhelming, so start small. Slow and steady wins the race.

Choose a part of your life that is easiest to make changes to first. Then make sure to celebrate your successes! Find an accountability partner to help you keep track of how well you are doing. They can celebrate with you when you hit milestones like 1 month of speaking positively about yourself. All these little things add up to big positivity. Have fun with it. You really are worth the changes you are making.

Gratitude unlocks the fullness of life. It turns what we have into enough, and more. It turns denial into acceptance, chaos to order, confusion to clarity. It can turn a meal into a feast, a house into a home, a stranger into a friend.

-Melody Beattie

Chapter 2

Gratitude

Gratitude is a genuine feeling of thankfulness. When you feel grateful for something your energy is raised to a very positive level. Gratitude is, in my opinion, the single most effective way to increase your positive energy. It is also a very simple tool to use.

The Gratitude Journal

Joy is what happens to us when we allow ourselves to recognize how good things really are.

- Marianne Williamson

I start and end every single day with gratitude. I list things, people and experiences that I am thankful for. Some days the list is harder to come up with than others. However, I am always able to come up with at least a few things. If you are a very negative person, or if you struggle with depression, this task may seem impossible. Thankfully I have found an easy technique that makes this Gratitude Journal a less intimidating activity.

First of all, it is really important to identify things that you really like or love. Make a list of all of the things you love to do, see and experience. Take a few days (yes, I did say days) to write a list of all of the things you find fun, pleasurable, amusing, inspiring, beautiful, special or interesting. Once you have this *Master List* you can simply read a few of the items off of it as your gratitude journal, on those days that you are feeling particularly low and can not seem to come up with anything off the top of your head. This master list can include anything that in even the smallest way brings you some measure of happiness.

For example, my master list includes things like sunsets, perfect temperature showers, massages, peppermint, laughing till I cry, my cats, the sound of my cat's purr, walking in the woods, snow crunching underfoot, butterflies, kissing...the list goes on, and on and on. For 4 pages single spaced and double sided I might add!

I compiled my list over a few days, adding to it as things popped into my head. I kept a small notebook with me at all times so I wouldn't forget anything. Then I put those random things down on the list. I used all 5 senses as they all have elements of joy in them. I listed all my favourite people (known and those I've never met), memories, places and experiences. Sometimes I read the list when I'm feeling down or discouraged. By the time I am halfway through I feel loads better! You will too. Once in a while you may need to redo the list, or add new things to it. This is also a great exercise for increasing your positivity.

Ok, back to the gratitude journal. I say things in my head or aloud now, but when I started this practice I made the habit of writing them down. There is something very therapeutic about putting things in writing. It also engages a big portion of your brain so that's a bonus!

I kept a book by my bed and every morning before I got up I would write at least 3 things I was thankful for. Some days I would start with simple things like my job, breathe in my lungs and food in my fridge. Some days I would have the same things to say as the previous day. Other days I got more creative. It really doesn't matter. There is no right or wrong way to do it.

This practice really sets your day up right. It opens you up to encountering more positive things. Then, at the end of the day, do the same thing. Come up with things specifically from that day if you can. Once this becomes a habit, you will be amazed at how much more consistently you feel positive.

Gratitude and the Law of Attraction
Gratitude is also helpful during the day. Every time you encounter something good, perhaps a beautiful blue sky or a person paying you a

compliment, say thank you to yourself (and the person who complimented you!). The more regularly you do this the more things you will notice you have to be thankful for. It is an easy process. When you find a great parking space, say thank you. When you get the advance green in a turning lane, say thank you. When you find a great deal on a pair of jeans – Thank you! It's so easy and it makes a huge difference in your overall well-being. I challenge you to do this for a week and see how much it affects your level of positivity.

Be thankful for all the positive interactions you have with people and you will find you have more and more positive interactions. This is the Law of Attraction at work. Think about it. You stub your toe when you get out of bed, then spill your morning coffee, then end up late for work...the world feels like is snowballing you doesn't it? That is because you gave so much energy into reacting to your stubbed toe! If instead you had laughed it off and turned your mind to gratitude, you would probably have found that your day went much smoother. At every moment you have the power of choice at your disposal. You have the power to turn your day around. Gratitude can help you do this.

Change the way you look at experiences. When you hit a bunch of red lights in a row perhaps that happens so that you avoid getting into an accident. The possibilities in life are endless. If you view the world as a place that is against you, or out to get you, undoubtedly you will encounter things that will support your belief system. It may come in the form of parking tickets, being late, or having a bad date. The reverse however, is also true. Thank goodness! If you have the belief that the world is *for* you, then all kinds of experiences will come to you in order to support your belief system. Perhaps it will come in the form of getting a great parking spot or an unexpected raise.

We truly are the creators of our own lives. Gratitude is a great tool to help you create a great life. You can even use gratitude in advance. Perhaps you have an interview in the morning. At night before bed, say to yourself 'Thank you that I will be confident and calm in my interview'. In the morning, reinforce that belief by saying 'Thank you that I am confident and calm'. You can also take this one step further and make the statement in the past tense "Thank you that I was so calm and confident in my interview today'. All of this is setting up your day in a positive way. Besides, according to Quantum Physics, time doesn't really exist anyways. So saying things in the past tense sends that positive energy to the situation when it was needed.

Nurturing Healthy Relationships

We all have friends and family members that we love. Sometimes we take these relationships for granted. Our lives get busy and we tend to see these people less and less. This is a common problem. So many people have too much on their plates these days, and it can be hard to find time to spend with our loved ones.

Our lives are all complicated but making time for those people who are important to us is crucial. These are the very people who help keep our positivity up! I guarantee that you are a person who aids in keeping their mood up as well. This is why it is so important to make time for our friends and family. It doesn't need to be a lot of time at once. Meeting for a brief walk or a coffee can do wonders for a friendship. Even a phone call out of the blue to someone who makes you smile can be a great mood enhancer. Think about how great you feel when you receive a call from a friend you haven't spoken to in a while. You feel awesome right? We all need these little pick-me-ups from time to time. They serve to nurture us.

When you take the time to call or see someone you care about, you are nurturing a special bond with that person. This is a healthy and necessary act. Make time at least once every couple of months to meet your friend in person if they live close enough. The more often you can connect the better.

You can even use things like Skype to connect when you are far away. Face time with a friend is far more beneficial than time on Facebook. Text and email are great time-savers but for forging a deep connection, face to face time matters.

Nurturing relationships definitely takes effort. It takes time and consideration. People are an integral part of our lives. The more you invest your time in healthy relationships the higher the benefit. This is why it is necessary to identify your most positive friends and family members. Spend most of your social time with these people. Limit the time you see people who are negative. They aren't worth investing as much of your time in when you are working so hard at raising your positivity. Invest in yourself this way. You are the most important person in your life. Choose who you spend your time with wisely and your positivity will always remain intact.

Gratitude is so important to your well-being. View life through a lens of gratitude and it will change your life. You will begin to see the beauty in details you never noticed before. You will also become better able to recognize the things that are worth spending your time, and perhaps your money on. You will be able to identify the people who are best for you to spend time with.

Gratitude opens up doors of opportunity, simply because you are thankful for the things you have now. Every time you nurture a good relationship, or take the time to notice things in your life that are special, you are sending a strong energetic message to the world. That message says that you are ready to have more of the good things, because you have admitted how thankful you are for all that you have now. Believe me, once you start embracing gratitude as a lifestyle, you will start to see more and more amazing things in your life.

A strong body makes the mind strong.

-Thomas Jefferson

Chapter 3

Exercise

For some, exercise can feel like the most boring thing in the world. What a chore! I was a Personal Trainer for 4 years so I've heard all the complaints you can throw at me. The bottom line is exercise is good for you. Not just physically either. If you want to increase your level of positivity, exercise is a surefire way to accomplish it. It floods your body with these amazing little feel good critters called endorphins. These are the same little guys that you get when you have an orgasm. You read it right. Orgasm! So unless you are having a tonne of sex, exercise is a pretty important thing to be doing to increase your positivity. If you do happen to be having sex aplenty, exercise will keep you in top form to keep it up. He he. No pun intended.

So now you *really* want to be exercising but you're thinking, how do I find a kind of exercise that I actually like? Well here's the thing, there are a lot of ways to exercise, and not all of them look spandex-clad and all competitive either. Walking, dancing, swimming, snowboarding, yoga, boogie boarding, bowling; these things all qualify as exercise. So finding something you like isn't really that hard. As long as you are off your butt and moving around a bit you can call it exercise. You can even exercise by playing on your Wii, if you're not cheating by tilting the controller with your hand that is.

If you want to do 'traditional' exercise in the gym and you are just starting out, I strongly suggest you hire a Personal Trainer for at least one session so they can set you up on a basic program. You can follow it and not be at risk of injuring yourself. I could tell you some serious horror stories of the poor form I've seen when newbies don't really know what they are doing. Yikes!

You may find it helpful to join a group or class at first. This way you can meet some people who are starting out too. You can use the buddy system and hold each other accountable. Make new friends and get active? What a bonus! There are so many kinds of fitness classes to choose from nowadays: step, cardio kickbox, Pilates, boot camp. The options are almost endless.

Looking for fun ways to exercise? Try Zumba or other dance style workouts. You are just boogieing it up so it doesn't *feel* like exercise the way running on a treadmill does. You can take up a dance form like Salsa or Hip-Hop too. Check out your local rec centre to see what they are offering. Sometimes I just make a playlist of great songs on my iPod and shake it in my living room. It's like that saying "Dance like no one is looking". If your living room isn't private enough for you, do it in the bedroom. If you are really feeling like having fun, dance naked!

Not all exercise is vigorous. Exercise can be a very relaxing and even a Spiritual activity too. Yoga, Tai Chi and Qi Gong are all practices that can be very grounding. There are many styles of classes available at local gyms and rec centers. Yoga styles abound and there is a style for every personality. These sorts of classes combine breath work with movement. This can be helpful if you feel like you are floundering and need to be more focused or centered. Yoga in particular can have a somewhat sedating effect if you choose a slower, restorative style. If you have trouble sleeping this may be a good choice for you.

As a special way to exercise, I sometimes like to drive to a wooded area with trails and walk in nature. This is like my church. I feel so connected to the earth. I can walk at a pretty fast pace and before I know it, a whole hour has past and I'm all sweaty. Fresh air is an added benefit. Walking is a great thing to do with friends too. It's a fabulous way to catch up and chat while getting you moving.

You can make dates and outings with friends active. Go bowling or ice skating. Strap on some roller blades or snowshoes and head outside. Hold a Wii or Kinnect games night and make sure everyone plays for real. Take up surfing or paddle boarding together. If your friends or your honey aren't into physical activity much, go online and find a walking or activity group. Meet some people who are interested in learning tennis or badminton. Speaking of which, the local rec centers and schools may hold drop-in sports nights for basketball, volleyball and other sports. You can drag your friend along or go and meet someone new.

The next time you have friends over for a BBQ why not organize a sports day like you had when you were a kid. You can make teams for hopscotch, crab walk, three legged race, potato sac races, wheelbarrow race, amoeba race and others. How fun would that be? Recapture your youth a little and I guarantee you will all end the night laughing your butts off. Wrap it all up with a game of Twister and you'll be the coolest host ever!

Make your next trip to the park or beach a heart-pumping trip. Bring along a football or baseball to toss around. Show off your mad Frisbee throwing skills. Bring badminton rackets and a birdie or two and show the kids how it's done. Grab the bocce or croquet set and play on a patch of grass. Lots of parks and beaches have volleyball nets set up in warm weather. Take advantage of them. Sure these may not all be the most fast paced activities, but you'll be moving a lot more than if you just sun-bathed the whole time!

Moderation

When it comes to starting an exercise program moderation is key. So many people jump in with both feet and end up falling flat. Start out slowly if you want to be successful and actually stick with it. Pick something you will enjoy and aim to do it once or twice a week at first. When you have done this consistently for a few weeks, then bump it up a little. Add a day at a time. Celebrate your successes along the way with little things like a new book or a pedicure. This will help reinforce the habit for you.

If you start going to a gym to lift weights or take a class, allow your body to adjust slowly. We tend to feel like we need to do it all or nothing but that isn't actually the best way to get started. Begin with the basics and once you are really comfortable with them you can move onto more intense and advanced things. Trust me, your body will thank you if you don't go too hard too fast. The old adage of no pain no gain is exactly that; old. The truth is that if you go hard too quickly, you really may hurt yourself and then you'll be less likely to get back at it the next week. This is about overall well-being, so focus on that instead of having an archaic 'go big or go home' attitude. That may work for some, but honestly I've rarely seen it work in the long run.

It is important to realize is that not all exercisers are created equally. This means that not all activities are going to suit every person equally. I'm talking physically and mentally here.

When I was in school I was horrible at block runs. I dreaded the days when we would have to run in gym class. Within minutes I would have a massive stitch in my side. I would have to walk the rest of the way and was often late for my next class. Add the fact that I was a bit smelly, having also missed having a shower, and let me tell you it was not a pretty picture. Put me in a pool though, and I could swim forever without really getting fatigued. I wasn't fast, but I had stamina in the water.

I am just not built for running, and I'm ok with that. I've found other things that do suit me. That's all that matters. I used to read in magazines that running was the best way to lean out and lose weight. That would frustrate me because I wasn't able to run. Now I realize that the best way for me to be my fittest is to do the things that I actually like doing. I'm able to stick to them because I don't feel like throwing up after. I also don't hurt so much afterwards that I need pain-killers to get through it either.

The payoff for doing what I am good at? It's easier. I enjoy myself. I stay motivated because

I'm not in pain. I've learned to listen to my body, to respect it, and the result is that I'm able to be in the best shape of my life without killing myself. You can too.

Focus on How You Feel, Not on the Scale

We have become overly obsessed with numbers in our culture. BMI, waist size, bra size, weight...it's gotten a bit ridiculous. The scale in particular is a really tough thing to look beyond. We live in a society that is totally focused on how much people weigh, particularly women. Sure weight matters but it is only one indicator of health. It doesn't tell you how healthy your heart is or your lungs. It can't tell you the difference between muscle and fat. It doesn't take into account bone density, organs, water. All it tells is the sum of your parts. Did you know that your weight can fluctuate as much as 10 pounds in a day! Not exactly an accurate way of keeping track of your health, or even your fitness progress for that matter!

There are far better ways to track your fitness level. You can keep a record of your heart rate at rest and during exercise. The numbers will most likely change as you become more fit. A marathon runner has a much lower resting heart rate than an obese couch potato. You can also track how you feel physically during workouts. If things start to feel easier, then it's probably time to make your workouts a bit more challenging.

Even these things aren't as important however, as how you feel emotionally. How do you feel before exercise? Do you feel low, grumpy, tired? How do you feel after exercise? Do you feel more positive? Do you feel proud of yourself? Perhaps you don't feel great immediately after exercise but overall you feel better from it. Some people feel more of a lasting benefit in their mood than an immediate one. Both results are great and neither is better than the other.

When I exercise I feel really proud of myself, because truthfully I'm kind of a lazy person. So when I get my butt off the couch and go do something active I feel better about myself. I feel better overall too because my body is in better shape when I am consistently being more active. I also tend to crave healthier foods. I feel more capable of accomplishing other things as well. I guess it's because exercise is not always easy to stick with. So when you do it, and make it a part of your life, you realize that you've succeeded at something. If you can do that, there are probably other things you can succeed at too. A sense of accomplishment can go a long way to increasing your positivity. Not only that, but there are real physiological changes that happen when we engage in active pursuits. We release those endorphins I mentioned before. You know, the 'orgasm' chemicals. They are physically in your body when you exercise, and they stick around for a while after you stop. Pretty cool huh?

Exercise also gives the added benefit of your body looking good. Yes, I realize that many people only exercise for this benefit. Regarding positivity, this is an added bonus, not the most important thing. Anyways, you will probably find that your clothes get a bit loose. You may even go down a pant size or two. Your clothes may look better on you too. This is because your muscles get more toned and defined when you exercise. I'll never forget the first time I realized I could see my triceps muscles on the back of my upper arm. It wasn't bulky or unattractive. It was just a bit more defined than before. It looked really good to me. Lean bodies show off clothes well and my shirt that day looked awesome.

So from now on, why not focus on how you feel instead of what that darn scale says. Your bones may be denser than you are aware of. Your muscle weighs more than your fat does. And water weighs quite a bit too. I haven't found any scale that tells you how much of each is in the final amount that it shows. If you must weigh yourself, make sure you are doing it for the right reasons: for reference, to make note of some change, or if you are part of a weekly weigh-in accountability group. I recommend that you only weigh yourself once a week or less. If you ever get on that scale and feel bad about yourself, stop stepping on it altogether. Increasing your positivity is crucial and anything that spurs a strong negative reaction, *especially* towards yourself, needs to be avoided at all costs. How you feel about yourself is immensely more important than what your body looks like or weighs.

The Great Outdoors

I can not say enough about the benefits of being active outside. I'm not talking about walking in the city here (though any amount of fresh air is great). I'm talking about getting out in nature. The sound of birds chirping, the sun on your face, the sound of wind in the trees...these things amp up our positivity almost immediately.

There is a park close to my home that I love to go for walks in. The trails are beautiful. When I enter that park I am transported to a place that is so peaceful. It is quiet, yet teeming with life. I get to hear all kinds of birds as I walk. I see squirrels running up and down the trees. Sometimes I'm even able to feed them some bird seed. Once in a while I see ducks in the creek. I absolutely love the sound of the water rushing downstream. I like the sound my feet make on the squishy ground after a hard rain. The leaves turn colour in the fall and look so pretty.

No matter what season it is the park looks amazing. I feel more alive there than anywhere. It is my little slice of heaven within the city. After a walk in the park I always feel rejuvenated. I get back in my car and feel lighter somehow. I always feel this way when I've spent time in nature. Nature has a real healing quality to it. Whether you are snowboarding on a mountain top, or swimming in a lake; nature draws you in. It takes hold of all of the worries and frustrations of the world and releases you from them, if only for a while.

If you don't know what to do outside, look online for local parks and lakes in your area. Beaches are great too. Anywhere that you can go where there are more trees than people is a great place to start. Reconnect with the earth in this way and I guarantee you will feel better for it.

There are all sorts of activities to do outside, regardless of the season. In the snow you can snowshoe, board, ski, toboggan, ice skate or have a snowball fight. In the sun you can swim, surf, paddleboard, kayak, skim board or jog. There are so many options. I've only scratched the surface. Find out what you love, and do it outdoors.

Remember the most important things about exercise are all about building your positivity. Make a list of active things you enjoy doing. Not sure what you like doing? Try something new. You are only limited by your own imagination and curiosity.

Once you start, make sure you listen to your body. Don't rush it. Be kind to yourself. Focus on how you feel above all else. If you feel good, then the activity is probably the right one for you. Get outside whenever possible. Have fun, be active and watch your level of positivity skyrocket!

All life is an experiment. The more experiments you make the better.

               -*Ralph Waldo Emerson*

Chapter 4

Hobbies

Embrace Your Inner Nerd

Everyone has different interests and talents. It is this variety that makes us all unique; special. Unfortunately, some people view certain interests and hobbies as lame or less cool than other things. In a word they are seen as Nerdy. I personally feel this is a pretty ignorant way to think. We are all so different, so it only makes sense that we would like different things. We can't all be psyched about football, video games and action movies. Life would be so boring if we did!

People may think that some interests are cooler than what you happen to be into, but really, who cares? I say embrace your inner nerd (or maybe your nerd has already come out of hiding a long time ago!). When I finally chose to stop hiding the nerdy things I liked, I found that my friends still liked me just fine. My brand of nerd is full of superhero movies (Wolverine is so cool!), karaoke, cookbooks, and Harry Potter. So what makes you happy?

To quote singer Sheryl Crow, "If it makes you happy, it can't be that bad". Seriously! Happiness is the right of all people. If you like things that your friends don't, I'm sure that you can find people who do. Join an online group. Groups exist online for every imaginable interest! Find a Meetup group, or if one doesn't exist in your area, create one.

Not sure of what you actually like? Try something new. There are hobbies and activities for every person on the planet. Collect stamps, study the stars, try your hand at sculpting. The variety of what you can do for fun is immense. Probably limitless.

Hobbies and passions are important. The people I know who don't have any real interests end up wasting their lives feeling bored. They watch TV to pass the time but they don't really enjoy it. That's not happiness. That's a shadow of what it is to thrive. With all that this amazing world has to offer, why live a bland life? That's not living at all.

Hobbies are mood boosters. If I'm feeling down, I pull out my paints and once I put paint to canvas I am transported to a place that is relaxed and beautiful. When I watch a silly cat video I find myself laughing, and I forget all about feeling depressed or bored. These particular things may not appeal to you, but when you engage in things that you like, your world will shift from a blasé place to one that makes you smile and feel alive.

It really is ridiculous to compare the coolness factor of one hobby or interest to another. What is important is to rate the level of happiness an activity brings you. If hockey rates a 1 out of 10 for you, leave it alone. If categorizing bugs rates 9 out of 10, then you've found a keeper. That's something really cool. So make a list of all the things you really like to do. Then when you are feeling bored or a little bit low, choose something from your list and run with it. You'll feel happier in no time!

Keep Busy

Hobbies and interests are helpful in elevating your positivity because they keep you busy. Boredom is one of the biggest downfalls of modern man. We have access to so much information but we sometimes forget to actually do things that captivate us. We get stuck watching mundane shows. We stay indoors far more often than is healthy. We have so many comforts and things that make life easier, but we don't always use our time wisely.

I'm not saying that you need to do things constantly to be happy. I am simply suggesting that watching countless hours of television, surfing the net endlessly and reading a bunch of fiction novels are not the only ways to spend your time. You have so many other options. Why settle for a mundane existence? Sure you may have your favourite TV shows that you love watching, but if you are honest with yourself, you will probably find that at least some of what you watch on TV, entertain yourself with on the net, and read in books is just a waste of time. People tend to find the 'best of what's on' instead of finding real gems to watch. This is pretty much the same as settling.

When you fall into this habit of settling, you are really just bored. Boredom is not a good emotion. Your positivity is neutral at best when you are bored. That isn't going to get you any happier. So get out and explore the world! All of those things you research on the internet actually exist for you to experience in real life. If you aren't in a position to travel, then explore your own city. Become a tourist in your own town. There is no excuse for being bored. Do something!

Boredom leads to things like mindless eating. Who the heck needs that? Hobbies and interests are great ways to fill your time without being bored. Make these things a regular part of your routine. Schedule time for them in your calendar. Make hobbies a habit instead of an occasional pursuit. Join a group or club that meets at regular times so you are always engaging in things that you love.

The busier you are, the more you will actually appreciate and benefit from the time you spend relaxing. Plus, if you are busy you can't really be bored. Your mind won't have time to think about anything but the tasks at hand.

Busy people are happy people. I'm not talking about workaholic busy. I'm talking about people who fill their spare time with things that they love doing. The people I know who are consistently doing things they enjoy are the happiest people I know.

Create Something

I have a brother who used to build and paint models. He was so good with his hands. His attention to detail was impressive. He enjoyed this quiet process so much. We always knew what to get him for gifts. Models kept him occupied and I think he found a sense of accomplishment in finishing them. He would display them in his room and bring them out to show them off when we had company.

I have never been great at detailed work; I just don't have the patience. But when I started painting I discovered what it was to create something. Now when I finish a painting I feel proud of myself. I feel like shouting to the world "Look what I made!" Creating something with your hands is an amazing expression of your inner self. It shows the world a small piece of you that it wouldn't normally see.

There are all sorts of ways to create something. You can start with the individual parts and put them together like my brother did, or you can start from scratch. You can use any medium you can think of. Clay sculpture, woodworking, drawing, painting, glass-blowing, metalwork, knitting. The list of options is as open as your imagination. Some people collect what others would call junk and then turn it into art. Other people decorate cakes. Whatever you think you would like doing, try it.

There are all sorts of books that have information on things you can create. You don't have to come up with something yourself. Learn from those who have done it before you, then put your own little spin on things. Go to the library and look up books on crafts. These aren't only for kids and grannies anymore. All sorts of people do crafts. I have a friend who makes all kinds of things. She makes her partner gifts for Valentine's Day that are so cool. She makes yoga mat bags and accessories and even ended up turning it into an online business! Are you starting to see the possibilities?

Recreation centers and schools often hold classes on crafts and hobbies. Local business may have workshops to attend as well. You can take a card-making class, learn the skill and then make it your own. I did this once with my step-mom. We had so much fun and our cards didn't look anything alike. The class was filled with women of all ages and backgrounds. It just goes to show that you never know who will be interested in the things that you are passionate about.

Check out websites for ideas too. I have found neat things to make on Pinterest and Facebook. There are all sorts of sites for inspiration. Do a search and find a site that looks interesting. Try your hand at some of the ideas you find and see what works for you. If you find the first thing you try is boring or frustrating, scrap it and move on to the next idea. This is not failure. You are just finding your own niche. There is no shame in experimenting with this. Eventually you will find something that wows you. If you already have a hobby, then books, classes and websites can help find ways to develop your skill. They can also give provide you with new ways of going about your hobby. Others may have tried techniques you have never even heard of before. They may also have tips for you to improve or simplify your creative process. Utilize other people's wisdom. You don't have to do it all on your own. There is not point in reinventing the wheel.

I was never very interested in traditional crafts but I have found lots of different hobbies and activities that I enjoy now. Some of them I only like doing with other people like card-making and ceramics; others I do on my own at home. I have recently discovered that when I have someone else over to paint with me, the paintings I create look very different than the ones I do when I'm alone. I guess the addition of another person taps into a different area of my creativity. That was a cool thing to discover. I like both ways of painting. Sometimes I just want to do it by myself, but now I know that it is an activity I can do with others without diminishing the final product.

Sometimes we find that hobbies keep us stuck inside. If you would rather do things outdoors maybe try bird-watching, gardening or photography. I used to have friends who did rock-balancing at the beach. You can look into sand or tree sculpture too. Some people make cleaning up the environment a hobby. There are clubs and organizations that devote their time to picking up garbage in parks. Whatever strikes your fancy, go with it.

You don't have to be the best at something to enjoy it either. Even if you are only making things for yourself that no one else sees, it is still a great experience. Your positivity will rise regardless of whether you have an audience or not. The more you do the thing you enjoy the better you will get at it anyways. Be proud of what you make and just love it because it is yours.

Fixing things is another great way to spend time if you are so inclined. I know guys who spend hours working on their cars, tinkering in the shop, working on tech items. They obviously get something out of it because they keep going back for more. Kill boredom by engaging in something that uses your hands. Every time you use your hands to create something or fix something, you are using that grey mass in your skull – your brain. Trust me; you want to keep using that brain of yours!

Try Something New

There's something liberating about not pretending.
Dare to embarrass yourself. Risk.

-Drew Barrymore

Taking a risk and trying something new can be a bit scary at first. This is actually a good thing for raising your positivity. Braveness is a mood elevator! When you put yourself out there and make yourself vulnerable you are choosing to be brave. That is a great way to live. Who would really choose to just be small and scared, if they were given the chance to live largely and be courageous? Most people would rather be brave.

The braveness factor is a curious thing. It can take a leap of faith to get started. Once you have jumped in with both feet and found that you can swim, you'll feel amazing. Decide on something you would really like to try and then just do it. Sure your heart may be pounding and you may feel terrified, but when you have actually done what you set out to do, your positivity will skyrocket.

What is something you have always wanted to do but never have? For me it was Zip-lining. I'm not great with heights so I was always scared to do this. I had heard that it was exhilarating and the views were beautiful and I really wanted to experience that. So one day, while in Mexico, I just decided to book the excursion. I went with a friend on a bus to this remote area, hooked on a harness, walked up a bunch stairs into the treetops and did it. Wow. That was probably the coolest thing I had done to date. It was fast. The air whipped my hair around and made my face flush. I hollered the first time and was so embarrassed. After that, I just couldn't get enough of it. The air was so fresh and the views were amazing.

I had a blast and I cannot wait to do it again. Plus, I had the added benefit of feeling like a freaking Champion! I felt like I had conquered the world. The feeling of freedom was intense. As I write this I am filled with the memory of that feeling. It is something that no one can ever take away from me.

I still struggle a bit with heights, but I know now that I can do anything because I faced my fear. I faced it and I laughed in its face. When you do that, your positivity will be through the roof. And every time you recall the memory of that, your happiness will increase. It's kind of the gift that keeps on giving. Try something new, especially if it is something that scares you a bit. I promise you that you will never be the same again.

Share Your Interests

Sharing your interests and hobbies is a really beneficial thing to do. When like-minded individuals gather, great things can happen. Ideas emerge, creativity opens up and possibilities come to the forefront. This creative environment can produce all sorts of cool new things.

Like I said earlier, when I paint with someone else my creations are different. The style is new and interesting. I get to tap into a part of myself that I just don't access when I'm alone. I have no idea why that is, but I'm happy to have found it out. I'm not actually working on the same painting as the other person, we are still doing individual work, but somehow the process is unique to that situation.

Sharing hobbies and interests with others also boosts your mood. Your passion becomes a social activity and gets you around other people. Pairing social time with hobbies is an easy way to really be happy. You are combining friendship with something you love, so your time with these people will always be a positive experience. If your current friends are not interested in taking part in your hobby, then find someone who will. Go online. There is a great website, Meetup.com where all sorts of groups are available to join. Every imaginable hobby and interest is represented there. If you can't find a group in your area for your particular hobby, then make a new one. I seriously doubt that you are the only person in your region that likes what you like. This may take you way out of your comfort zone. Remember how I felt when I faced my fear of heights when I went zip-lining? You can feel the same way when you create a group and get others out to engage in your activity.

Actually, the first Meetup group I went to was started by a woman who was an introvert. She was shy, quiet and timid. She created a social meetup group for single women in her area because she was having trouble making friends. I imagine that starting the group must have been really scary for her. Going to the first outing was a bit daunting for me, and I'm an extrovert! For her it must have been really terrifying. I'll bet that she was pretty proud of herself afterwards though. She had faced a fear head-on and ended up meeting some pretty cool people in the process. You can too.

Find what you love and do it. When you regularly take time to pursue your interests you are honouring yourself in a deep way. Your positivity will most certainly increase. You'll be having fun and that is all that really matters in life. Ditch the boredom. Do what you love and love what you do. You will be happier, more positive and a more well-rounded person.

Kudos to you if you conquer a fear or two along the way.

If I knew I was going to live this long, I'd have taken better care of myself.

-Mickey Mantle

Chapter 5

Therapies

My belief is that when the body is in a relaxed state, it is able to heal itself. The human body is incredibly effective at performing self-healing. Unfortunately, we have moved away from this innate ability. We have instead fallen into the practice of relying on external, artificial means of coping with illness and disease. We have stopped listening to our bodies and allowing it to do what it knows to do, in order to keep us well. Our bodies are miracles of science that we choose to ignore!

After a really awful personal experience with the 'health care system' in Canada, I found myself on a plethora of medications for depression and anxiety. The result? I was a freaking Zombie! My pupils were so dilated I freaked myself out every time I looked in the mirror. I was emotionally stunted. My senses were over-stimulated. My body was weak. I had virtually no immune system. I developed a sweet tooth that was out of control. I could barely walk a block without being completely exhausted. My sleep pattern was out of whack. Basically I was a total mess. Health care system my ass!

So I slowly weaned myself off of all the medications I was taking. Then I started researching natural remedies and techniques to reduce stress. I also looked into natural alternatives I could use to help with my depression and anxiety. I have been off of medications since June of 2008 and have never looked back. I did take medication when I had a manic episode in 2010 for a brief period. For me, this is the way medications are meant to be used. Briefly, to help get over an issue that is not correcting itself.

I am *not* a medical professional and do not recommend you stop taking medications without some sort of professional guidance. I know that there are some conditions that really do need prescription medications. I also know that a lot of conditions can do with less medication or none at all if other things are used to reduce stress, and keep the body at optimum health.

When I was doing all of this research, I was looking in a lot of different books and websites to access all the information. I've decided to include some of the items I found in this book. This is not an exhaustive list. Perhaps I'll make one for a future book. I hope that you try some of these methods and remedies. You will be better for it. They are all wonderful and I highly recommend them all. Please realize that not every technique will work for every person. We are so very unique that some things just work better for some people. I'm confident that at least one of these things will help raise your level of positivity.

Acupuncture

Acupuncture is a great therapy for reducing anxiety and depression. It is also a fabulous way to treat physical pain, which can be a symptom of depression. I first went to an Acupuncturist when I was coming off of the medications I was on. The initial appointment lasted almost 2 hours. The practitioner did a very thorough exam of my tongue, pulses, skin, eyes, ears and lymph nodes. I had wanted help with my anxiety but he discovered that I had more pressing issues that needed to be addressed first. My liver and lymph nodes near my underarms were greatly inflamed. He had me feel both areas with my hands and explained what they should feel like. I was especially shocked at how much I could feel my lymph nodes.

Lymph nodes are part of your Lymphatic System, or Immune System. When these become blocked or inflamed, the body can not effectively do its job of getting rid of toxins and keeping you healthy. I had been on so many prescription drugs that my immune system and liver were overloaded. My body wasn't able to deal with the toxic load. I allowed the Acupuncturist to work on this issue before dealing with my anxiety and I am so glad that I did. Within 2 weeks my liver had returned to its normal size and I could no longer feel the inflammation in my lymph nodes. I was surprised at how quickly the changes occurred. I found that I had more energy after these sessions and was sleeping better as well.

Acupuncture is based on the principle that we have *energy meridians* in our body that allow our life-force or 'Chi' energy to flow through us. When these energy meridians become blocked or our Chi becomes unbalanced, practitioners can clear these blockages and imbalances by inserting tiny needles at precise points on the body. This technique can help with anxiety, depression, grief, PMS, menopause, phobias, pain relief and a slew of other disorders, illnesses and issues.

I happen to have a severe phobia of needles, but as I was desperate to find a natural way to cope with my anxiety, I was willing to try Acupuncture. I was relieved to find that most of the needles were painless (I actually didn't feel the majority of them at all!). There were a few that were a bit painful for a second or two when they were first inserted. A few others hurt a tiny bit awhile after they had been inserted. I would sometimes feel one of them get hot, or the area around it would throb. This apparently means that a big blockage is being cleared. The results I experienced were amazing and I always felt so relaxed after my sessions. I often felt blissful for hours after I left the office. I have come to love Acupuncture and I go fairly regularly to keep my energy flowing well. I would definitely say that it helps my positivity remain at a high level. It could be a great option for you and I highly recommend you try it. It also happens to be reasonably priced so that's an added bonus.

Reiki

If you have never had the chance to experience Reiki you are in for a treat. It is a form of energy healing that is based on similar principles as

Acupuncture. It can be described as a *facilitated relaxation technique*. When the body is relaxed, it is able to heal. Did you know that almost all cell regeneration and repair happens while we are deeply asleep? This is because the body can finally work on repairing and healing itself when it is resting. When we are awake and dealing with everything we encounter during the day, our bodies are busy performing all its other functions. It just doesn't have time to work on healing. That's why it isn't wise to eat a big meal before bedtime. When you do, you are forcing the body to work at digesting food instead of healing and regenerating!

So back to Reiki. Imagine how happy your worker-bee cells will be if you allow them to focus on some of their healing and restorative tasks during the day. This is what Reiki does. In a typical session, you lie on a table and just relax. A Reiki practitioner places their hands in various positions on or above your body to help facilitate energy flow. Some people feel nothing at all during these sessions. Others may feel heat in areas, or cold, vibrations, twitches and many other sensations. All of this is completely normal. During my first Reiki session I didn't really feel anything at all. I just seemed to swallow a lot and at one point let out an odd noise from my throat. I did feel very calm and relaxed.

It was after the session that I noticed a change. I had bought a painting easel and supplies kit at Costco some months before. I hadn't actually painted yet though. I was sort of scared to put paint to canvas. I was apprehensive because I didn't want to mess it up and I had no experience with art except a bit of art therapy in the hospital. After that first Reiki session I felt this great desire to paint. It was the oddest thing! The thought just came to me at the end of the session when the practitioner asked me for feedback. I didn't paint my first painting that day. I painted it the day after. Now I love painting abstract paintings. Reiki cleared me of negative energy that was holding me back through fear!

Reiki is one of the most amazing modalities that I have found. I actually got my Level 3 practitioner certification in Usui Reiki last year. I love Reiki. I use it for myself all the time, and for my cats. If you are interested in finding a Reiki practitioner check out the resource section at the back of this book. You may also want to look into where local Reiki Shares are in your area. These are wonderful get-togethers with people who use Reiki already, or want to experience it for the first time. I love Reiki Shares. They are very supportive and welcoming groups of people that provide a safe environment for newcomers. Reiki is awesome. Book a session or attend a Reiki Share and expect great things.

Massage

Who doesn't enjoy a massage? I can not think of a faster way to deeply relax the physical body. Massage is a wonderful method of relaxation and stress reduction. Many benefit plans cover massages if they are performed by a Registered Massage Therapist (RMT). The cool thing is, lots of great spas have RMT's on staff. You can book a Relaxation Massage with an RMT at a spa, and have it covered by your work benefits!

If you have never been to a spa for any treatment before, you really will love it. The entire experience is quite lovely. The ones I have been to have all kinds of luxurious perks, ranging from yummy treats, wine, flavoured water, magazines, a lounge to hang out in and saunas. You can spend hours there just soaking up the cozy, relaxed atmosphere. It's fun to go with a couple of girlfriends. They also usually offer couples massages. So book a massage and get that stress out of those muscles!

Chiropractic

Ok, I know that a lot of people consider going to a Chiropractor anything but relaxing. It can seem like a very scary thing. I used to agree with them. Who the heck would want to volunteer to have their neck or back be cracked? Fortunately, I had the opportunity to work at a Chiropractor's office. My opinion changed very quickly. I had my first *Chiropractic*

Adjustment and I found relief in my neck and shoulders immediately.

Your spine has a natural shape. Through physical stresses, traumas, poor and lazy posture, we alter this shape. This causes our energy flow to become blocked. Remember that Acupuncture helps to unblock your Chi energy? Chiropractic adjustments do the same thing for your spine. Our spines become *subluxated* or misaligned. These subluxations cause pain, discomfort as well as other issues including migraines.

A Chiropractor manually adjusts your spine by applying pressure in specific positions on your body to help release the subluxations. The snap crackle pop that you hear during an adjustment is simply a release of gases within your joints. It is completely safe and highly effective at pain relief.

Keep in mind that one session will not cure you of anything. Your muscles have gotten used to holding your spine in place. They don't know that the position they have been holding it in is an unnatural one. It will take some time to train them to hold the new position. Most clients at the office I worked at started out with 2-3 sessions per week for a couple of weeks. Then they went down to 1-2 sessions a week, then every 2 weeks, every 3 weeks and eventually once per month. If you do go to a Chiropractor please be open to this kind of schedule. You really will reap the benefits if you commit to it. You will probably find that you begin sleeping better and feel more comfortable with day to day activities. Try it. Your spine will thank you.

Art Therapy

When I was in the hospital I met a woman by the name of Jane. She was an Occupational Therapist. I am eternally indebted to her. She was a kind, soft-spoken woman who was incredibly patient and wise. She introduced me to art therapy.

I didn't taken art in high school and had limited experience with it before that. It never occurred to me to try it after I graduated. I never imagined I would like it. In the hospital Jane held workshops for the patients. I liked going to these classes to learn different things. One of them was a painting class. She had us paint our feelings and ideas on paper. It was really fun. It was also a very effective form of therapy.

Sometimes when we are struggling personally, it is difficult to put how we feel into words. This is especially true when we are dealing with things like depression and grief. When words escape us, we can communicate through art. I don't mean that others will necessarily look at what we have painted and know what we are feeling. I mean that this can be a beautiful way of expressing emotion when you don't feel you are able to talk about it.

You can paint abstract or realistic paintings. Neither is better than the other. There is no right or wrong in art. It is simply you expressing yourself in colour. You can paint how you feel, where you are at inside. You can paint your fears. You can paint your dreams. This method is limitless. You can paint whatever you want, however you want.

I painted my pathway to health while I was in the hospital. When I left and started feeling more healthy I painted what that felt like. I've come to love painting and I do it as a hobby now. Whenever I feel low, I know that I can take out my paints and express myself in a safe manner through my art. Painting isn't the only way to use art as therapy. You can colour with crayons. Remember how much fun you had doing this when you were a kid? Play around with artistic crafts. Try your hand at pastels. Draw on the sidewalk with chalk. Make origami. Take a clay sculpting class. The possibilities are endless. Who says these things are only for kids? I think that if we all embraced our inner child a bit, we would be much happier, positive people. I even bought a used Spirograph on eBay to play with. Every once in a while I pull it out and it always makes me smile.

Counseling

Over the course of my life I have seen counselors for a variety of reasons. I have gone on my own and with family members. I find having a neutral person to talk to refreshing. When you vent to a friend or family member, they are on your side. It's kind of their job to be. They see your point of view; empathize with you. Sure that can make you feel validated, but sometimes having someone with no emotional attachment to you can be very helpful.

Counselors are neutral parties. They listen well and give appropriate feedback. They are able to give you perspective. When you find yourself emotionally charged around a person or experience, it can be difficult to see clearly. You may feel that there is only one way to look at it, or that you are completely right. This is when a counselor can help you move forward in a healthy way. They can make suggestions for you to try. They ask questions that help you look more deeply at the problem. They can also help you find solutions that you probably wouldn't find on your own.

If you are experiencing things that you need help sorting out, go see a counselor. The first one you see may not suit you so be open to seeing more than one to find one that fits your needs. I have gone to both men and women. Through openness and exploration, I have found a great counselor that I go to periodically when the need arises. Ask friends, coworkers and family members for referrals. You can also ask your medical doctor for names of reputable psychologists in your area. I recommend you try counseling if you are dealing with issues and not finding any real solutions to your problems. The neutral perspective a counselor can offer is a really great thing.

Hypnotherapy

After I had weaned myself off all the medications I had been put on for depression and anxiety I found that I felt stuck. I didn't know how to progress any further forward. I was attending regular counseling sessions and, although they were helpful, I needed to find some way to take the next step toward a healthier mindset.

The psychologist I was counseling with suggested I try hypnotherapy. She knew a new hypnotherapist in the area who was getting her required practicum hours for certification. She referred me to her as she knew this woman had reduced rates for her practicum hours, and I was on a tight budget at the time.

I admit I was hesitant to try hypnotherapy. I had seen the parlor tricks that hypnotists pull on their volunteers at carnivals. I really didn't know what I thought of hypnotherapy. I had come to trust my psychologist though, so I booked an appointment.

The hypnotherapist was very nice. She explained what hypnotherapy was and what it wasn't. She told me that the subconscious mind was powerful. She helped me understand that when a person is hypnotized, they are safe. You can not be forced to do something under hypnosis that you would not willingly do under normal circumstances. We discussed my concerns and she answered all of my questions respectfully. So I decided to give it a try.

The process of being hypnotized was actually really cool. I felt very relaxed. Once I was 'under' my subconscious was able to be communicated with directly. It was so interesting. She would ask me questions and I answered them with ease. I didn't have to really think at all, the answers were automatic and true. Over a series of sessions I was able to deal with some deep-seeded issues I didn't realize I even had. It was illuminating and freeing at the same time.

I have been to two hypnotherapists and both helped me with different things. Sometimes I find myself 'stuck' again. When I do, I book a hypnotherapy appointment. These sessions help me identify underlying causes of my feelings, habits, and perspectives. Sometimes the root cause of things is a huge surprise! Every time I identify the real reason I am feeling or behaving a certain way, I am able to really look at it, and re-evaluate it. I have found every time that once I do that, the issue dissolves. It doesn't have a hold on me anymore because the reason I *thought* I was struggling isn't even true. Freedom can be found in the strangest of ways.

Remember, all of these therapies are useful when you are feeling negative or low. They are even more useful at elevating and maintaining a positive, happy feeling. If you use some of these things as a means of preventing those slumps we are all susceptible to, you will find that they happen a lot less often. That is the aim after all. Do all that you can to keep stress at a minimum. Focus on enjoying life more, and you will.

To me, if life boils down to one thing, it's movement. To live is to keep moving.

-Jerry Seinfeld

Chapter 6

Movement and Music

One of the most wonderful things about life is the ability to move. Movement comes in many forms, ranging from the necessary to the frivolous. There are forms of movement, such as Yoga, Qi Gong and Tai Chi that are highly beneficial to us when we want to raise our positivity.

Yoga

I first tried yoga many years ago. I had read a review of a yoga video in a magazine and was curious to check it out for myself. I went to the video store (back when they were still popular) and rented a copy of the tape. I waited until my family was in bed before trying it, because from the cover it looked like I would be putting myself in some pretty compromising positions. I didn't want to risk the embarrassment of having my brothers see me attempting them.

The video was a bit difficult even though I was in excellent shape. I found that I had no flexibility to speak of and was surprised at how my body reacted to the positions (called postures). I had never been overly bendy, even as a child. So I knew that this form of exercise was going to be good for me. I used to watch gymnasts on television in awe of how they could move and stretch. I'll admit I have always been jealous of friends who could do the splits.

I started doing the yoga routine every second day for a few weeks. My body became accustomed to the moves quickly and I felt so good doing them. My muscles were challenged in a new and exciting way. I became more flexible sooner than I would ever have hoped. A fabulous side benefit was that my posture greatly improved. I hadn't expected that at all.

The practice of yoga was grounding and almost meditative at times. I found myself focusing so much on my form and on my breathing that it got me completely out of my head while I was doing it. I loved how relaxed and invigorated I felt after each session.

Since first using that video tape to learn yoga, I have experimented with other styles. Some suited me better than others. I found that some styles were relaxing and great for evenings; other styles were great for waking me up and energizing me.

Here is a general run-down of the styles I have tried:

Hatha – a general form of yoga that is slow-paced and great for beginners.

Vinyasa – also called Flow Yoga; times the breath to the movement and tends to be vigorous. I recommend this for intermediate levels and above.

Ashtanga – also called Power Yoga; fast-paced, intense and vigorous. It is a great workout for intermediate or advanced participants. The same movements are performed in the same order each time.

Iyengar – poses are held for long periods. Props are encouraged to bring the body into proper alignment. I found this a good class as a beginner.

Restorative – very relaxed and slow form; props are used and poses held for several minutes to allow the body to naturally deepen the stretch. This was great for before bed. I was able to do this style as a beginner.

There are other forms of yoga worth checking out; these are just the ones I have personal experience with. Find a class in your area and try it out. See what works for you. There is probably a form of yoga that is perfect for your needs. Yoga is a great way to release stress from your muscles. Any way that you can tap into deep relaxation and release tension is a good thing. Give yoga a try, you may just find it is the best thing you ever do.

Qigong

I learned about Qigong (pronounced chee-gong) when I was weaning myself off of prescription drugs. My body was overloaded and I was looking for natural ways to de-stress. I read about the practice of Qigong online and in a book on Traditional Chinese Medicine and was intrigued by it. I found a Qigong DVD at the local library.

The practice is a form of movement that focuses on breathing. When you perform Qigong you promote your Chi energy flow, much like in Reiki and Acupuncture. It is actually a form of therapy, but as it is also a form of movement. I decided it made sense to put it in this chapter.

Like yoga, Qigong can be energizing or relaxing. Some movements and types of breathing used are intense and best performed during the day. Other forms of breathe work and movements are slow and therapeutic; great for unwinding before bed. I really enjoy Qigong in the morning. It wakes me up and energizes me for my day. I took a class at the rec centre by my house for a while. I found that taking a class helped me understand the movements and types of breathing better, as some of it can be confusing on video if you are new to it. You may find Qigong is a fabulous daily practice. I recommend you check it out.

Dance

You've gotta dance like there's nobody watching...

- William W. Purkey

Dance is sublime. When you allow your body to sway to the rhythm of music you enter a world that is pure and wonderful. Pulsing to the beat of a drum, moving along with a guitar riff; dance transforms you. It makes you feel one with the music. It doesn't matter if you have no natural rhythm at all. You just feel good doing it.

I love to dance. I have no formal training, I just move the way my body wants to when my favourite song comes on. Sometimes I go out with my girlfriends and dance the night away. Other times I just feel like dancing by myself at home, so I put on some fun music and shake it.

It makes me feel alive and definitely improves my mood.

There are so many styles of dance. If you are keen to learn a particular form, there are all kinds of classes available. Dance studios and recreation centers offer classes on styles like ballroom, Latin, hip hop, belly dance, bhangra and others. I tried belly dance at a girls' night once. It was hilarious! We had so much fun and the instructor was great. We got to use finger cymbals and scarves as props and we jiggled our way through an hour of choreography. It was a great workout. I loved it.

Some people don't like to dance. It may be because they aren't comfortable in their own skin, or perhaps they feel awkward in their movements. Thankfully, if you are one of these people, you can still enjoy dance. There are many local dance studios and clubs that put on shows for the public. Live vicariously through the people on stage. Live dance is fabulous to watch. You get to see beautiful movement to music, and the training the performers have had is clearly evident. Some colleges and universities also put on dance recitals, as do high schools. Do a little research to find shows in your area. There may even be dance festivals near you. You can also go to bigger events such as the ballet.

Music

What can I say about music? It is a universal language. Everyone can appreciate music. You don't even have to understand the words. There doesn't even have to be words! I have a love affair with music. I love to sing, I dabble in percussion and dancing is one of my favourite things to do.

Music is a unique thing; a gift. It can amplify your mood and it can shift it too. Use the right kind of music at the right time and it can ward off depression and grief. Use the wrong kind and it can further your journey into the depths of despair. Music in a word is *powerful.*

There are so many styles of music I doubt it is possible to come up with an exhaustive list. Every genre contains sub-genres. If you haven't found at least one style of music that you like, you probably just need to do more searching.

Within every genre there are examples of positive music and negative music. I suggest that you spend the majority of your time listening to the positive selections. Remember, words are powerful. Combined with music, words become *immensely* powerful. I caution you to take that combination very seriously. If you are at all inclined to raise the positivity in your life, these details matter.

Dr. Masaru Emoto, a Japanese water scientist, did an amazing study on the effects of words, and music on water crystals. He found that when water was exposed to classical music or positive words, the crystals looked beautiful, intricate and perfect. When water was exposed to hateful words or dark music such as heavy metal, the crystals became deformed and horrible looking.

You can see the results of his study online and in his published works. I have included them in the resource section of this book. When I saw the pictures from his study I was shocked.

When you consider that your body is made up of 60% or more of water, this study is really enlightening! Your brain is made up of about 75% or more water. So words and music, have a physical effect on you, even if you don't think they do. That is why it is so crucial that you choose music wisely.

If you like heavy metal, it isn't necessarily all bad. Again, words *and* music affect us. There are no studies that I could find that focused on the effects of dark sounding music that had positive words. Neither could I find studies that focus on the effects of nice sounding music with negative words (there are many examples of this too!). I personally think that as long as the way a song makes you *feel* is good, then it is probably just that. Feeling is the key. If you honestly feel fabulous then you are doing something right.

When it comes to music, it is important to pay attention to the lyrics. If you don't know what the song is saying you have no way of knowing if it is affecting you positively or negatively at a subconscious level. You can't go on sound alone.

There are so many songs that sound upbeat and fun but the lyrics may be about very negative topics such as suicide, hate, crime, cheating, lying, stealing; you get the point I'm sure. Musicians use lyrics to get their point across. It is the easiest way for them to affect their listeners and bring them around to their point of view. Sometimes their view may not be the kind of viewpoint that benefits you. If you are serious about becoming a positive, happy person, be mindful of what you listen to.

Classical Music

If you don't already listen to classical music I recommend you check it out. Classical music can be therapeutic. It helps the mind relax and can even help you sleep better. Studies have shown that listening to classical music while studying increases the amount of information you retain. Pretty powerful stuff!

I love classical music. I listen to it before I paint. I find that it helps me tap into my creative side. It soothes me on a deep level. I also use classical music to calm me, as a way to prepare for meditation and anything else that requires me to focus. As there are many different styles of classical, you are bound to find some pieces that you enjoy. When I need to do a big clean of my home, I sometimes opt for loud, boisterous classical music instead of pop, rock or dance music; especially when I'm sorting papers. This way I am still pumped up and motivated by the music, but I'm not distracted by the words.

You may be new to classical music, but I imagine you have heard some in movies and cartoons at the very least. If you aren't sure where to start, check out movie scores, the big composers such as Beethoven and Mozart, or use a search engine to find popular pieces online. I have included some options to try in the resource section at the back of this book as well. Go explore this genre and fall in love with it as I have.

Percussion

A lot of people think that all percussion instruments are drums. This is incorrect. A percussion instrument is anything that is struck to make a noise. Bells, rattles, xylophones and drums are all forms of percussion. One of my brothers is a drummer. I used to love playing on his drum set when I was younger. He would let me play when I was frustrated or angry and it really helped me hammer away my emotions. It was an effective way to release my pent-up feelings. I wasn't very good at playing to music but that wasn't really the point for me.

Since those days of banging on his drum set, I have discovered a love of percussion. I have friends who meet once a month for a drum circle. This may sound a bit weird, but it is actually really cool. They sit around a fire in the backyard and just start drumming. There is no song, it is just rhythm. It evolves into a beautiful noise after awhile. Sometimes other percussion instruments are used too. I have gone to these circles a couple of times. I found them interesting and oddly comforting.

If you are interested in trying percussion, pick up a cheap drum or rattle and just play with it. Bongo drums are common for people to start with. You can bang on them to the beat of some music at first. Then you can try your hand at creating your own music. You may have drum circles in your area as well. Search for groups online to see what is available to you.

Playlists

While we are on the topic of music, I may as well mention using playlists. If you have an mp3 player or even just music on your computer, you can make playlists. There are tutorials online to learn how to do this, or just enlist the help of a friend. It is easy to make a playlist.

I have playlists that are specifically for increasing my positivity. I find all kinds of uplifting songs and put them all in one playlist regardless of the genres. I keep this playlist on my phone and in my car at all times so I can have it close by. I listen to it when I get ready for work, and before I go out to see friends and family. I listen to it when I'm feeling down, and for when I just want to raise my positivity a bit.

Using playlists in this way supercharges your positivity before you go out into the world. When you are already feeling great before you encounter others, the odds are you will be better able to cope with whatever comes your way. If you know you are going to be dealing with emotional vampires or people who are a bit challenging to be around, prepare yourself with a playlist that is designed to make you feel great. This is like putting on armour before a battle. Protect yourself.

I listen to a positive playlist when I drive. That way, I'm feeling happy and if I run into traffic or bad drivers, I'm barely affected by it. The music is keeping my mood in check. I rarely react badly to a situation when I'm listening to upbeat, encouraging music. If I do react, I don't internalize it and allow negativity to overcome me. Can you see how using playlists can help keep you positive? If you don't have much appropriate music for a positivity playlist, find some by searching online or going to the music store and exploring.

I realize that others may find this playlist of yours a bit silly. When I first started listening to more positive, happy, uplifting music, it was met with mixed reviews. I chose to listen to it only when I was alone, or with people who didn't judge me for it. Nowadays I just don't give a damn what anyone thinks. When you are starting to make changes in your life, anything you do to protect yourself from negativity is a totally okay. If you need to keep some things a secret it is understandable. Just do what feels right for you.

So there you have it. Movement and music are your allies. Use them to increase your positivity whenever you need a pick-me-up. These are great tools to have in your arsenal. Have fun with it. Who knows? You may even find your inner dancer or rock star!

Kind words may be short and easy to speak, but their echoes are truly endless.

-Mother Teresa

Chapter 7

Words

According to the Law of Attraction, our thoughts become things. We create our reality through thoughts and words. Every word you say is an extension of a thought you have already had. Confused yet? I used to be too. Let me simplify it for you.

We have already established that words are powerful. Remember that Japanese scientist with the water crystal experiment? That is real. He found tangible evidence to support the idea that words affect us physically. So what does this mean for the average, everyday Joe and Jane? Well here's the thing; you get to choose your thoughts, your words, and your feelings and therefore *you* are in control of your life. Sound good? It can be.

Words can be used to create an amazing world that you love. They can also be used improperly to create a world full of sadness and struggle. You get to choose which life you want. Words can either bless or curse. I'm not talking about religion here. This is simply fact. Read the following words and concentrate on how they make you feel. What imagery is attached to them for you? What memories do they bring up?

Hate.   Sadness.   Fear.   Anger.
Cruelty. Jealousy.   Bitch.   Jerk.
Devastation.

All of those words bring up negative feelings and images for people. Now repeat the exercise for the next selection of words.

Happy.   Elated. Joyful. Whimsical.
Love.   Bliss.   Victory. Hilarious.
Energized.

They feel different don't they? That is the power
of words. They connect us to past memories
and present experiences. They also affect our
future life. When you continually say negative
words regarding your situations, experiences,
friends, family and yourself, imagine the affect it
is having on you. You need to become mindful
of what you are saying so that you can shift your
energy from positive to negative. This can take
time, so be patient with yourself during this
process.

Blessing and Cursing

I have created an exercise for myself that may
help you begin to use positive words more
often. Make a list of your closest friends. Beside
each name, say what you would like to bless
them with if you were able to. For example, if
you have a friend named Carl who is struggling
at work, write "I bless Carl with job satisfaction

and success". Do this for as many people as you like. You don't need to limit yourself to one thing per person either. Do as much as you want.

Once you are done, read it aloud. When I do this exercise I read it aloud at least once a day for a few weeks. This gets me in the mindset of using positive and encouraging language. I believe it also sends good intentions as energy to the people I'm blessing. It's kind of a form of prayer. Keep your intention positive and for the person's highest good. No harm can come from this practice.

When you have done this for a while, I suggest you then do it for yourself. Think of things you would like to improve in your own life. Are you happy in all areas of your life right now? Probably not; there is always room for improvement. Write down blessing statements for yourself such as "I bless myself with improved health and vitality". Write as much as you want for as many areas as you need. Then start saying them aloud to yourself at least once a day. I find it easiest to do this before bed.

When you do this as a regular practice you will begin to feel happier in those areas of your life.

Blessings are great mood boosters. When you are blessing your friends, family and yourself, you can't help but feel good about life in general. Cursing however, has the opposite affect. You probably don't think you are in the habit of cursing people (unless they cut you off in traffic perhaps). Unfortunately, all those words you say to people that are mean, biting, petty and cruel have an effect, not just on them, but on yourself as well. Every time you say a negative word about someone or something, that word originated in your thoughts. That means that negativity has been in your head and regardless of what it is aimed at, you get burned by it in the process.

Negative energy and positive energy are opposites. You can not be filled with one and also filled with the other. So if you are focusing much of your attention and time on negativity, positive energy simply cannot flourish within you. You need to focus the majority of your energy on positive things. It's that simple.

You may think that monitoring your thoughts and words will be tiring and boring. This isn't actually true. You can use your feelings as an indicator tool. If you *feel* good, you are thinking good. Simple right? Focus on how you feel about the things you are doing in your life. If anything brings up a red flag for you, consider making some changes.

Every day choose to bless instead of curse. Pay random compliments to people you meet. Talk about the things that you are excited about. Change the topic when someone is complaining. You determine what you focus on. Choose wisely and watch your positivity soar.

Negative Self-Talk

I know I have already touched on this before but I believe it warrants further focus. How you talk to, and about yourself is crucial to your well-being. Even the most minor words, when used consistently, can have a big impact.

I used to refer to myself as stupid and silly a lot. After I did something clumsily or without really thinking, I would say "I'm so stupid" or

"How silly of me". I never realized just how often I was doing this until a friend of mine mentioned it. She told me that I said things like that about myself all of the time. From that day on, I made sure I paid attention to my self-talk. Sure enough I found that I said things of that nature constantly. I made a commitment to myself to stop it.

This was a daunting task at first. Thankfully I remembered the Elastic Band technique! I would thwack my wrist with an elastic band every time I caught myself using negative self-talk. My wrist hurt badly for the first few days. The exercise sure worked fast! I didn't want to have welts on my wrist so I just stopped talking smack about myself. Now I rarely find myself doing it.

You can use something I like to call Positive Self-Statements to help you as well. These are not the same as *affirmations*. They are simply factual sentences about yourself in the present tense. Find a few things you truly like about yourself and write them down. If you can't think of any, ask a friend for examples to use. When I first did this, I chose one thing about my physical self (my smile) and three things about my personality and abilities. For example, if you are a skilled artist, you can write "I create beautiful art that people love". If you regularly have friends confide in you, write "I am a good listener". Write your statements on a cue card. Make a couple of copies so you can put them in different places such as your car, bathroom and jacket pocket. Read these to yourself or aloud as often as possible.

When you hear something often enough, it becomes true to you. Your brain makes the connection between the statement you are saying and the feeling it conveys. Eventually these words will be strong mood boosters for you. When they become like old friends, create some new ones. Do this whenever you find yourself in a slump. It will help remind you of the things that make you a wonderful person.

Books
Obviously books are filled with words. And as we have already established the importance of

words in our lives, I thought it prudent to discuss books. What you read has an affect on you. Just as the lyrics in songs are important to keep track of, so are the kinds of books you read. If you only read books that are filled with negative imagery, you are basically choosing to fill your emotional tank with bad fuel.

I used to love crime novels. The more graphic they described the crime scenes the more I loved reading them. If you have balance between positive and negative reading, then the odd crime novel is probably just fine to read. I didn't have that balance. I only read gruesome books and the majority of what I watched on TV were crime dramas. I eventually connected my disturbed sleep with what I was watching and reading. I quit crime-based entertainment completely for a while until I could find balance. Now I have a much healthier balance in what I read and watch.

Reading fiction can be a great thing for your psychological health. When you read interesting, creative books your mind has a chance to relax. It has time to de-stress. There is a reason that people say they can get lost in a book. Reading engaging material gets you out of your head for a while. Like I've said before, that can be a very good thing indeed.

There are also an abundance of non-fiction books worth reading. I have read some great biographies of successful and positive people. They often have great information for overcoming obstacles. Books on success can also be beneficial. These books usually provide some insight on the psychology of success. I have found many interesting notes on being happier within success books. I like to read self-help books too. They are often filled with interesting ways to raise your positivity.

Books hold a wealth of information. You can find so many valuable books at your local library and bookstores. Look for books on topics that interest you. Find books about your hobbies. Read what you love. If you feel good reading it, then it is a good book for you.

Keeping a Journal

I have already mentioned keeping a Gratitude journal. Now I want to tell you about the value of keeping an every day journal. Some people call them a diary. Whatever you call it, these notebooks can help you in a big way.

Sometimes you won't have time to get together with a friend to discuss your day. In these times, a journal can be a sort of surrogate friend. Write all of your feelings and experiences down as a way of purging your day. Write without stopping so that you aren't attaching too much emotion to the words. This is especially helpful in removing negativity from you. When you start to feel strongly about what you are writing, stop. Put your pen down. Take a deep breathe and remind yourself of things you are thankful for. This will shift your energy back to positive. If you feel you are able to continue writing without becoming frustrated or upset, then start writing again. If you know you are too wound up, simply put the journal away. This technique helps release negativity that you have attached to experiences and people you encountered during your day. After you are finished this exercise, do some deep breathing. As you inhale, focus on filling yourself with positive, happy feelings. As you exhale, picture all negative emotions leaving your body.

I do not recommend you read your journals. Some people find this therapeutic but I have found more often than not, that I just end up re-living the negative memories. If you want to keep a journal about positive experiences, then have a separate book for this. Keep the negative away from the positive. Read the happy one as often as you like. Once a year I usually discard my journals. I have ripped them up, shredded them, simply thrown them in the trash, and even burned them. All these methods served the purpose of purging me of any lingering negativity from within those pages. I especially enjoyed burning my journal, but this isn't always a safe option.

There is another method of journaling that I have dappled in that you may enjoy. It is called *Art Journaling*. Basically you draw, paint or colour your emotions and experiences. This is really fun and puts a new spin on recording your struggles and successes. There are books designed especially for this. If you use regular books, paint will bleed through the paper. Go to a bookstore or art supplies store to find an art journal. Some of these books have prompts to get you started such as "use colour to express the prominent feeling of the day" or "draw your favourite experience today". If you are new to this type of journaling, these prompts can be really helpful.

Singing

So many people sing that I knew I had to include a bit of information on this topic. People sing in their cars. They sing in the shower. They sing while getting ready for work. People sing in church. Singing is a big part of life for many people. I sing a lot. I love it. Karaoke is one of my favourite things to do.

So why is singing included in this book, apart from the music section you ask? Well, singing uses words. Singing also often includes some pretty strong emotions. Think of your favourite songs. When you are belting them out, you are putting an abundance of emotion and focus into the words you are singing. So, if you are singing at the top of your lungs along with a band that is known for its harsh lyrics, you are doing yourself a disservice. The act of singing passionately amplifies whatever the mood of the song. If it isn't a happy or uplifting song, you are focusing a tonne of energy on the wrong thing.

I know some of you will not like to hear this. Music is a personal thing. Remember though, that your mood is everything. Negativity breeds negativity. There is no way around that simple fact. If you are serious about raising your positivity then you will make sure you are being careful about what you listen to. You will also be extra careful of what you sing.

Words said or sung with feeling are powerful. When you sing passionately, you are basically putting a giant magnifying glass to the emotion that song conveys. Sing the wrong kind of song, and all your hard work will be for nothing. So if you are going to sing, choose songs that have positive or neutral lyrics.

Words are powerful. Don't ever forget that. The words you choose to use in your daily life can have a profound impact on your world. Choose them wisely. Choose to bless and not to curse. Use words to encourage others. Most importantly, use words to encourage yourself. Build yourself up instead of beating yourself down. Your positivity will rise swiftly with every positive word that leaves your lips.

Happiness is when what you say, what you think, and what you do are in harmony.

-Mohatma Gandhi

The soul should always stand ajar. Ready to welcome the ecstatic experience.

- Emily Dickinson

Chapter 8

Creative Techniques

There are some ways of reducing stress that are not exactly therapies. They are techniques that help the body and the mind relax. I have found many different, and sometimes unconventional, ways of lowering stress in my life. Sometimes finding what works for you takes time and a little creativity. Keep an open mind regarding the following techniques. You never know where and how you will find relief.

Deep Breathing

Obviously we all breathe constantly. Did you know though, that few of us actually breathe deeply? We use only the top third of our lungs to breathe most of the time. This is a bad habit the majority of people have formed due to stress in their lives. Think of a baby sleeping. A baby automatically breathes from its belly during sleep. Those deep breaths make its belly rise up and lower down in a very obvious pattern. That is how we are meant to breathe. Unfortunately most of us breathe from our chest. Our shoulders tend to rise with the inhale and our chest rises and pushes out. Our bellies barely move. This indicates that we are not really breathing deeply at all. It is truly beneficial to use deeper breathing at least as a daily practice. This allows more oxygen to get into our cells. Our cells all need lots of oxygen to function.

Allow me to reintroduce you to the Belly Breath. If you practice this daily, perhaps as a nighttime ritual, your body will thank you for it. It is a fabulous way to reduce stress and release tension from your body and your mind. It can actually be a form of meditation for you, as you focus on your breathing and nothing else.

For a basic form of deep breathing follow these steps:

1.) Lie on your back, preferably without a pillow at first.
2.) Place your hands on your abdomen with your fingertips touching.
3.) Take a deep, slow breath in. Notice if your hands move apart slightly. Exhale slowly, allowing your fingers to touch again.
4.) Continue this slow breathing in for a count of 4 and out for a count of 4.
5.) Focus on your breathing. Feel the flow of air moving in and out.

If your fingertips did not move apart at all, focus on your breath, and push your belly out as you inhale. Allow it to collapse as you exhale. Keep doing this until you feel it become more natural, no longer forced. Visualize your breath flowing deep into your belly and then out through your nose or mouth. This may take some practice so don't get discouraged if you don't figure it out right away. You probably haven't breathed like this in a very long time. Your body and mind are retraining right now. Be patient with yourself. You'll get it when you are ready.

There are many forms of deep breathing that you can play around with. I have included some websites in the resource section of this book that have some great information on this. Try different breathing styles to see which method you like the best. This is a personal thing and you may find another form more effective than the one I have described. I promise not to be offended. These techniques are all wonderful stress relievers. Anything that reduces stress and tension really help to boost mood. Make deep breathing a regular part of your routine and your positivity will definitely increase.

Zen Gardens

You may have seen miniature Zen Gardens in people's homes at some point. A Zen Garden is basically a tiny sand box with a rake and some stones in it. These things are really relaxing to play with and can be pretty fun too. All you do is remove the stones, take the rake and draw designs in the sand. Swirl it around in a smooth motion. When you feel like you are done raking, place the stones in the sand wherever you like. This is a simple creative process that gets you out of your head for a while. We could all use some timeout from our heads right?

This may seem like a silly exercise but think about how much fun kids have in sandboxes. Remember how much fun it was to make a sandcastle at the beach? There is something very appealing about moving and molding sand. You can find Zen Gardens at some bookstores, in Asian markets and online. Check out the resource section at the back of the book for some options.

If you are not interested in using sand, I have also found a form of water therapy very relaxing too. Put your hands in a container of hot or warm water. Move your hands around slowly; rhythmically swirling the water. Allow water to drip from your fingers. Focus on the feeling of the water on your skin. You can place rocks in the water as well and hold and rub them during this exercise. Allow your body to relax and your mind to become calm as you watch your hands moving in the water. Combine this with some deep breathing if you like. Slowly moving your hands, almost like they are dancing is an interesting way to raise your positive energy.

Emotional Check-In

This technique doesn't actually raise your positivity directly. It serves as a kind of emotional barometer. Emotional Check-In, when used regularly, will help you identify how you feel. This is super important because when you are able to identify and label your feelings, you have the power to change them if you need to. When you realize the freedom this brings you, doing this exercise regularly will become very important to you.

An Emotional Check-In focuses on 5 main areas:

1.) Spiritual
2.) Mental
3.) Emotional
4.) Physical
5.) Social

I often add a 6th category *Overall* as well. Ask yourself "How am I feeling Spiritually?" (If you are not a Spiritual person, you can either disregard this one, or think of it as your deepest feelings.) When you ask this question, you may feel supported, removed, angry, distant, bored, stimulated...the options are as varied as emotions themselves. No feeling is *bad* either. Feelings are all valid and serve a purpose. Some are just more positive than others. If you are feeling crappy spiritually, this just tells you that you need to focus on your Spirituality a bit so you can raise that feeling to one that is positive.

Ask yourself "How do I feel Mentally?" This has to do with your brain folks. If work is stressing you out or you are tired and feeling unfocussed then your mental health is something worth focusing on. I sometimes feel mentally foggy, bored, calm, alert, stretched, taxed, even confused. Identify the feeling. If it isn't a feeling that feels particularly good to you, then use this information to your benefit. Find out what is causing you to feel this way and then make some changes.

Ok, so how are you feeling Emotionally? Are you all over the map? Do you feel depressed, anxious, worried, bored? Do you feel happy, elated, balanced or blissful? These feelings are the equivalent of your positivity rating. Make a note of them and if you think they need some improving, do some of the things in this book to increase your positivity.

How does your physical body feel? Are you tired? Restless? Tense? Do you feel energized? Perhaps you feel sexy. Maybe you feel vibrant and alive. If you are feeling anything negatively in your physical body, get a good night sleep and make sure you are getting some sort of exercise. You may need to eat more healthily or drink more water. Limit your alcohol and caffeine intake. Monitor your physical feelings and deal with things that need to be dealt with. This isn't rocket science here. You probably already know what you need to be doing, so just do it.

How you feel Socially is really important too. This has to do with your interactions with your coworkers, family and friends. It has to do with how often you see other people and the kinds of things you do when you are with them. Monitor this closely and you will probably find out if you have any *Emotional Vampires* in your life (see chapter 1).

How you feel towards other people in your life strongly affects you. When you are constantly fighting with friends and family, your mood will undoubtedly be lower than is optimal. If you are having lots of fun with others, your mood will be high. Sometimes you may become over-socialized. Other times you may be too isolated. These can both be negative things. Balance is the key here, so make sure that you are making time for yourself as well as others. When I do my check-ins, I often mention to myself that I am feeling socially happy or sad about a certain person or group. This helps me truly identify any underlying factors in my relationships that are affecting my positivity. Great tool huh?

You may have noticed that I mention boredom a lot. That's because boredom is never a good thing if you want to be positive. Feeling bored is actually a pretty negative emotion. It implied that your life is bland, blah, uninteresting, unexciting. Who the heck wants their life to be like that? If you find that you are feeling bored in any area of the Emotional Check-In, you need to work on that area! Read the chapter on hobbies for some ideas to create a more satisfying life. If you are bored mentally, you may benefit from a more challenging job or from taking a class. Reading non-fiction or

watching documentaries and informative shows
may help as well.

Identify your *Overall* feeling as well. You
may be Spiritually open, Mentally Alert,
Emotionally content, Physically tired and
Socially bored. What is your overall mood
though? Maybe your overall mood is actually
happy. Sometimes breaking it down into these
little pieces can be a bit too complex in reading
the barometer of your mood. As long as your
overall emotion is a positive one, you can relax.
Just make a point of working on any negativity
when you have the time.

I hope you make this Emotional Check-In
technique a part of your daily life. It is often
used in programs like Alcoholics Anonymous
and for good reason. This technique is highly
effective in reconnecting with our feelings. So
often we squelch things, push them under the
carpet and forget about them. All this does is
cause them to fester and grow in an
undercurrent. At some point you will have to
deal with how you feel anyways, so why not do

it on a daily basis before any big issues develop?

I use this technique throughout the day. Sure there are days and even weeks that I fall out of the habit, but for the most part I use it on a daily basis. It has been an incredibly powerful tool for me. When you identify any negative feelings you have, you are able to improve those feelings by taking action. Positivity becomes a choice. How's that for a possibility?

Earthing

There is a relatively new movement in natural health called *Earthing*. Basically this is the act of placing your bare feet on natural ground and allowing yourself to connect with the Earth's energy. This may sound like hokum but it is actually an effective way to decompress. We all have energy fields and so does the Earth.

Go to a park or a beach or even your own backyard and take off your shoes and socks. Stand on the grass or sand and really focus on the feeling of it against your feet. Wiggle your toes a bit. This can be a very grounding exercise. We are so often wearing shoes and socks that we don't really experience the connection to nature this way. We rarely have bare feet outdoors unless we are at the beach, and even then we aren't focusing on the feeling of our feet on the ground.

When we do this kind of activity we pull away from the stresses of the day. It is a way for us to just *be*. In a society where people are expected to be doing things all of the time, it is a great relief to just *be* without *doing*. It is like a breath of fresh air. It provides a break from routine.

You can also sit on the ground if you like, and run your hands through the grass or sand. Remember when you did this sort of thing as a child? Again, this is reconnecting you to the things you innately knew when you were young. We used to play on the grass all of the time, looking for 4-leaf clover, watching bugs, daydreaming. Somewhere along the way, we forgot what it was like to just be. Take some time to explore how that feels again. I'm willing to bet that you'll feel happier for it.

These creative techniques are all very helpful. As you explore different methods of stress reduction, keep an open mind. It is also a good idea to try different things at different times. I have found that some things will be helpful for different kinds of stress or emotional overload. Not every technique will work every time. Some techniques may not work for you at all. Try different things until you build a toolbox of sorts. Do this and you will always have a variety of options when you need them most.

Have nothing in your houses that you do not know to be useful or believe to be beautiful.

-William Morris

Chapter 9

Internal and External Environments

Everything we digest and everything we surround ourselves with has consequences. Some things are far better for us than others when it comes to our level of positivity. If you want to be truly happy the majority of the time you must make sure that all things within and without are harmonious.

Nutrition

Let food be thy medicine and medicine be thy food.

- Hippocrates

When it comes to nutrition there are a few things you need to know. Strict diets are out. Instead, focus on balanced nutrition that allows for some healthy indulgences. Stick to food that is as close to nature intended most of the time and you'll be just fine.

There are three types of macronutrients that you have probably heard about: protein, fat and carbohydrates. Your body requires all three of these to function optimally. If you restrict any one of these you will be headed for trouble. Avoid products that say things like low-fat and low-carb because these processed foods are filled with toxic chemicals designed to make you addicted to them. Natural is always better.

Fat may start with the letter 'F' but it is not related to that other F-word. Fat is actually your friend. It fills you up and makes food taste good. It is essential in the absorption of vitamins and minerals. It helps lubricate joints and provides energy for cells. If you eat low-fat foods you are doing your body a great injustice. Fat from coconuts, avocados, olives and nuts are great Vegetarian sources. Animal sources like butter, ghee, meat and fish are also very healthy. Even bacon is great for you when it is organic. Watch for sodium levels in cured meats though. Moderation is key for these items. Eat a bit of fat at every meal and you will be satisfied for much longer than if you skip it.

Protein is responsible for many processes within the human body. All vegetables and fruit contain some protein. Obviously meat, eggs and fish do as well. Grains contain protein but are harder for the body to digest. You may not know this, but there is something called *bioavailability* which is important. Basically some foods may contain a high level of protein but the body can't easily access them. Eggs are a fairly easy protein source to digest as is fish. Lentils are possibly one of the easiest vegan sources. If you do eat grains, stay away from wheat as it is very hard on the body. Sprouted grains such as barley are much easier to process. Most people find brown rice and quinoa easy on the system too. Eat a moderate amount of protein at every meal. Your body can only process so much protein at a time so don't overdo it. A serving size is about the palm of your hand.

Carbohydrates. This seems to be a dirty word these days. This is unfortunate because your brain requires good quality carbohydrate to function. If you want proof of this just go and watch a body-building competition. The diet of most of the competitors the week leading up to the event is extremely low-carb. When asked to turn to the left many competitors stay facing straight or even turned to the right! Their brains are so depleted of carbohydrate that they actually become dumb. What a sad state of affairs.

All vegetables, fruit, grains and legumes contain carbohydrates. The starchy carbohydrates are the most difficult to digest. These include foods such as potatoes, beans and any wheat-based and other grain-based products such as pasta and bread. I recommend you stick to fresh or frozen fruits and vegetables as much as possible.

The easiest way to make sure you are getting all the vitamins and minerals you need is to eat a variety of colours. Red peppers and strawberries; oranges and winter squash; lemons and summer squash; leafy greens and avocado; eggplant and blueberries. These are examples of how easy it is to eat from the rainbow of produce available. If you are willing to try new foods you will find that the variety available is immense.

Eat a mixture of raw and cooked vegetables. Some nutrients are easier to access raw; some cooked. Eat more vegetables than fruit, as sugar content is usually higher in fruit. Think of fruit as nature's candy. Moderation is wise. It is easier on the body when you eat fruit on it's own as it digests very quickly.

When it comes to positivity, eating well can go a long way. A body that is well-fueled just feels better than one that is running on junk food. Fast food is an oxymoron. It isn't food at all. It is just junk fuel for an amazing body. Feed yourself well and your body will thank you. A well-fueled body sleeps better and is more energetic when awake. Your immune system will be much stronger and more efficient if you eat healthily too. That means less colds and flu.

A lot of people focus on calorie counting and portion control. I personally believe we are meant to enjoy our food. Focusing on numbers detracts from that enjoyment. Instead, fill your plate with lots of veggies and some good quality meat, fish or lentils. Use lots of herbs and spices to flavour your food.

Chew thoroughly and savour each bite. Enjoy your food. Eat slowly so you will be able to tell when you have eaten enough. When you eat, make it a time to relax. Don't watch TV or work at your desk while you eat. Take time to taste your food and your level of positivity will be much higher. As an added bonus your stress level will be lower too.

Remember that it is okay to indulge once in a while. Have some ice cream or chocolate. Just make sure you really savour it. Eat it slowly to make sure that it is really worth your while.

When we cherish our indulgences and really enjoy them they are much sweeter.

Supplements

Many people take vitamin supplements. If you are concerned about nutritional deficiencies I advise you to instead take a whole foods supplement. These are usually available at grocery stores. If you cannot find them there, take a trip to your local health food store. These supplements (often found in powdered form) are easier for the body to use than regular vitamin tablets. A lot of vitamins you take end up being expensive urine.

There are other supplements that can be beneficial. If you are a vegetarian or vegan it is important to take a B12 supplement as it is mostly found in animal products. Find a *sublingual* tablet form that dissolves under our tongue, as these are easier for your body to process. Vegetarians may also want to supplement Omega 3. Vitamin D is important for people who do not get much outdoor time. The sun (even on cloudy days) is the best source of

Vitamin D, but it doesn't hurt to have a bit extra in pill form on those dreary winter days. If you are wondering what other kinds of supplements you need it is wise to go see a Holistic Nutritionist or perhaps a Naturopath.

Notice I didn't recommend a dietician or medical doctor. I personally feel that the education a Holistic Nutritionist and Naturopath receive is more balanced in nutrition. Dieticians and medical doctors only look at the Canadian or American food guide as a standard. This is very limiting and biased in my opinion. I may have opened a can of worms saying that but the advice I have received regarding nutrition from conventional doctors has been lacking and limited.

Another great source of information on nutritional supplements, especially natural herbs and supplements is your local health food store. The staff at these stores are educated on many natural products that are often safer and more effective than common prescription remedies. Go have a chat with one of these people and find out all sorts of things that may help meet your personal needs.

Supplements are wonderful but it is important that you do your homework. Ask questions and make sure you find out if there are any contraindications with medications or supplements you are already taking. Your health is your responsibility, so educate yourself accordingly.

Sun and Sun Lamps

There are few things that feel better than sun on skin. The warmth feels so nice on those first days of spring, especially after a long fall and winter season. Sunshine brightens everyone's mood instantly. The first sunny days turn us all into little sunflowers. It is a common sight to see people turn their faces upward to feel the sun's rays on their cheeks.

Sunshine is a wonderful thing. It provides Vitamin D for our bodies. It also holds promise of summer bounty in the form of lovely summer produce. Berries and all manner of fruit abound when the sun comes out. When you are eating seasonally, spring and summer are special times of treasure.

Unfortunately many areas of the world do not get as much sunshine as people would like. For some the lack of sun can wreak havoc on their well-being. There is even something called Seasonal Affective Disorder (SAD). People who struggle with this find themselves prone to bouts of depression during lengthy periods without sun. If you are one of these people, there is relief. Sun Lamps are a great invention. They mimic daylight and allow the body to produce adequate amounts of Vitamin D right in the comfort of your home. It only takes about thirty minutes a day to alleviate symptoms of SAD. You can find these special lamps at some drugstores and grocery stores. You can also find them online.

Décor and Colour

It may surprise you but colour is very important to mood. What colour you wear can have a direct effect on your emotions. The colours you surround yourself with also make a difference in how you feel about the world. Not convinced? Some prisons paint the walls of isolation rooms pink because it helps calm the inmates down!

So what colour is the right colour to wear? It depends on what you want to accomplish that day. If you are feeling a bit down then choose a bright, cheery colour such as yellow or orange. If you are feeling stressed or erratic wear blue or green. These colours tend to be calming. Feeling feisty? Put on a ruby red. You'll feel like you can take on the world. Colour is an easy way to convey how you are feeling, or how you want to feel, to the world. It is a subtle but effective form of communication. There is a whole science behind the effects of colour.

How do you choose what colour to paint or decorate with? Well, think of the activity you will do in each room. In a bathroom you may want to use yellow to help you feel awake in the morning. In the bedroom you may want to use calming colours like blue or green; neutral browns so that you can feel relaxed when you go to bed. If you have an office where you need to tap into your creative side, purple may be a good option. There are lots of books on *colour theory* available. Do some research before you do any painting. You may want to add small, decorative items in a certain colour before you commit to paint.

Candles

Sometimes you need a bit of mood lighting to make you feel good. Lighting candles and turning down the lights can be very relaxing. You can listen to classical music, sip a glass of wine and really unwind. Candles can be mesmerizing. Watching the flame flicker is an instant mood soother.

I love lighting candles in my home at night. Storms and power-outages are obvious excuses to do this, but you can do it just because you feel like it too. I sometimes colour in the dim light of candles. Sometimes I just sit and watch the flickering flames. Candles create a positive space to reminisce and to dream of things you want to do someday. Light candles when you are in the bath for a more inviting atmosphere. They are sure to help you reduce stress.

Baths

Having a hot bath at the end of a long, stressful day provides deep relief. Your muscles hold lots of tension and a bath helps soothe them instantly. Add some bath salts and your bath becomes an oasis.

Soaking in a bath can be a special experience. Listen to beautiful music. Light some candles. Sip a warm beverage. All these things, when combined with a hot bath, add up to a spa experience at home. You can read in the bath. You can add bubbles and sit listening to them pop.

A bath is one of those simple pleasures in life. Take time to pamper yourself with a warm bath and soothe the tension of the day away. Do it right with all the trimmings and you are sure to really enjoy yourself.

You have a lot of control over your internal and external environments. What you eat, wear and surround yourself with is all up to you. If you choose to treat yourself well, your positivity will improve greatly. Eat healthy, supplement wisely and make sure you get some sunlight as often as possible. Surround yourself with beautiful things in the form of colourful décor and plants. Take the time to pamper yourself a bit with candles and a hot bath. All of these little things can really make a difference in your mood. Do these things. You deserve it.

Happiness is a choice that requires effort at times.

-Aeschylus

Chapter 9

Soulful Remedies

I have already mentioned the most effective ways that I know to raise your positivity and be a happier person. There are a few more things I would like to mention now. These particular things may be fairly obvious to some of you, but I feel they are worth mentioning. Sometimes when you are experiencing a dark period in your life, it pays to have a list of go-to activities that can help you feel better. The ideas in this chapter will nourish your soul. They focus on your inner world while working on your outer world. These remedies can benefit you on a deep level if you are open to them.

Hugs

Now I know this isn't exactly rocket science, but physical contact is a huge help in elevating mood. A good, solid hug is one of the best things you can give someone who is feeling down. Getting a hug from someone you love provides the warmest of feelings. It doesn't have to be romantic for it to be effective either.

When people hug out of genuine affection, they actually transfer their energy to each other. This shared energy charges you up similarly to the way Earthing does. This is a highly effective way to make both parties feel wonderful. It is an easy way to let someone you care about know that you value them and love them.

Think about it. How do you feel when you receive a hug? It's a great feeling right? When you haven't seen a friend for a while and they pull you into their arms and really hug you, it feels like they are clinging to you out of a deep need. This feels amazing. Without any words, a hug conveys those deep emotions of love. I can think of nothing else that does this as effectively as a hug. So the next time you see a friend or family member that you've been missing, give them the best hug you have ever given. You'll make their day and you'll feel awesome too.

Pets

Animals are very special. When we open up our homes to a pet it is wonderful thing. Pets fill us with joy and are great companions. They often pick up on our moods and stick by us when we need company.

Growing up I was fortunate to have a variety of pets. Some were more fun than others but looking back, they all were valuable to me at the time. Even the family Guinea Pigs were sweet additions to our home. Dogs of course were more active and playful. Cats were a source of entertainment. Birds were sometimes noisy but they had their merits as well.

As an adult I have the pleasure of owning two wildly amusing cats. One is tiny and the other is massive. They can be tedious and demanding at times but they are my constant companions. I love them so much. I cannot imagine what life will be like when they are gone.

When I am sad or scared my pets are always at my side. On those days when I am sick and stuck in bed, they usually never leave my bedroom. They show me unconditional love and affection. Animals are like that. They are happy to just be in your company.

Some hospitals actually use 'pet therapy' as a way to help patients deal with depression. Petting an animal alleviates emotional pain. When I feel stressed out I reach for one of my cats and just pet them. They purr and I feel instantly better. If you are able to provide a happy home to a pet I recommend you do.

Laughter

I honestly think it's the thing I like most, to laugh. It cures a multitude of ills.

- Audrey Hepburn

This may seem like the most obvious thing to do when you feel down but unfortunately when you are truly sad, laughter doesn't come easily. Because this is so, it is a good idea to keep some things on hand that make you laugh. If you have a variety of items available you are more likely to use them to cheer yourself up.

Gather a collection of funny movies. Choose ones that you know you will enjoy watching over and over. Then grab yourself some funny pictures. There are loads available on the internet. Many websites exist simply to make you laugh. Keep them handy.

Let friends and family know what your favourite funny things are so that they can share them with you too. Laughing with others is always more fun than doing it alone. You tend to laugh harder with company too. Laugh as often as possible. It will keep your mood high and you'll just feel great doing it.

Success Journal

Celebrate your successes. Even the small ones. Every time you celebrate something you are proud of doing it creates a positively charged feeling within you. Keep track of things you did well. Make a note of accomplishments. This is really important. The more you acknowledge things you do right, the more likely you are to continue doing them.

Buy a small notebook and use it to write down your daily successes. These don't have to be things that others think of a success. This is a personal thing for your eyes only. If you regularly struggle to clean your home, write down all of the little things you do during the day to keep your place tidy. I used to really struggle with this so I started patting myself on the back every time I *did* clean and before I knew it, cleaning became a habit for me. This is called positive reinforcement. Celebrate your little successes and you may just find that bigger successes follow.

Every night before you go to bed write down at least three successes. They can be as simple as remembering to take off your makeup, or doing a load of laundry. They can also be big things like paying off a credit card. Whatever feels like a success to you, write it down. No successful activity is too tiny.

Be proud of what you have accomplished. When you hit milestones really celebrate by telling other people. Reward yourself with a new book or a dinner out. You deserve to celebrate when you have done something that you are proud of.

Random Acts of Kindness

Think of the last time a stranger paid you a compliment. Maybe they told you they liked your sweater. It probably felt pretty fabulous didn't it? Now think of how you felt the last time you did something kind for someone else out of the blue. You felt great then too didn't you?

Performing random acts of kindness is one of the simplest ways you can boost your own mood. This is another form of energy exchange. When you do something nice for someone else you are actively making the world a better place to live in.

Smile at a stranger as you pass them on the street. Better yet, say hello to them. Help an elderly person with their groceries. Open the door for someone. There are countless ways we can be kind to others. I often pay compliments to people I don't know. I find something nice to say and then I just say it. I know that it has a lasting effect on that person and it costs me nothing at all.

Take every opportunity to be kind. Make it a habit and you'll probably find that more nice things start happening to you as well. This is the Law of Attraction again. I guarantee that at the very least you will have more things to say at night in your Gratitude Journal. You'll feel good about yourself too. When you make kindness a habit, you become a better version of yourself. That is the best thing to be.

Forgiveness

Forgiveness is a gift you give yourself.

-Suzanne Somers

Forgiveness. It can be the hardest pill to swallow. When someone has wronged us we tend to feel angry and bitter towards them. Hold anger in you heart for long enough and it becomes a grudge you are holding. Grudges are unhealthy and they hurt no one more than you.

I learned the hard way that forgiveness is necessary if you want to be happy. You cannot be filled with negativity and positivity at the same time. One always dominates. Negativity usually wins in this game unless we choose not to let it.

If you want to truly be positive and happy you need to start letting go of any anger and bitterness you are harbouring for others. Make a list of all the people who have done you wrong. It may be a long list so take your time and be thorough.

Next, write out all of the things that each person has done to hurt you. Overwhelmed yet? This is a process. Set some time aside to do this task well. Dig in your heels and go deep with this exercise. Grab some tissue if you need it. Tears have healing qualities so don't hold them in. They actually release stress hormones from your body so cry your eyes out if you want to.

Once you have your 'record of wrongs' take a good look at each entry. Write down what part you played in the event, if any. Be honest with yourself. More often than not, both you and the person you are mad at are partly to blame for what happened. This is going to be a humbling experience. Don't be afraid of that. In the long run it will provide a great sense of freedom.

If you realize that you need to pay some apologies, do so soon. Let the person know that you are sorry. Making amends, though never comfortable, frees you from negativity. If you don't know the person anymore or feel it would be unwise for you to talk to them about the issue, write them a letter. You don't need to mail it. The act of writing it out can be enough to release the negative emotions.

For the people and events you have left over, you have a couple of options to proceed with. You can choose to see their perspective. Put yourself in their shoes. See if you can imagine what they were thinking at the time.

Really see their side of things. If you do this and find that you are able to let your anger go you are finished with that event.

The other way you can deal with it is to burn the papers. As you burn them speak release over the events. Tell God or the universe or even just yourself that you forgive the person and you release them from your anger. Meditate on this for a while. Don't rush it. Say it aloud to yourself and mean it. Take deep cleansing breaths and visualize the anger leaving you with every exhale.

Forgiveness is not an easy thing. It takes effort and commitment. It is one of the best things you can do for yourself. Forgiveness frees you of resentment, bitterness, sadness and anger. It allows you to look back on experiences with new perspective. Look on them with love and affection. See them as valuable lessons learned. You don't have to feel badly about your past. Forgive and let live. While you are at, forgive yourself too. You deserve as much as anyone else.

Meditation

For many people the idea of meditation is confusing. It is such an abstract idea. Talk to someone who regularly meditates and you may find that they don't really sound like they are even speaking English when they describe what it feels like.

Meditation doesn't have to be complicated. It is simply a calming of the mind. Our minds tend to be on overdrive much of the time. Meditating helps get your thoughts under control.

A simple way to begin meditating is to sit upright on a cushion. Cross your legs if it is comfortable. Make sure the room is quiet and without distraction. Close your eyes and focus on your breathing. Feel the air flow into your body and then out again. Just focus on your breathing.

If your thoughts wander that is totally okay. The goal is not perfection. Rather the goal is to quiet the mind, not into total silence, but to slow it down. Do this for five minutes a day at first. As you get used to it, increase the amount of time and maybe do it twice a day.

Play with this a bit. You can focus on a word or statement. You can focus on an image. You can focus on anything you like. Just allow your mind to be calm and undistracted for a bit of time. This will help you feel calmer during the day. It may also help you sleep better. Meditation can be a wonderful way to increase positivity in your life. I have listed some websites and books in the resource section that may be helpful to you.

Makeovers

One of the quickest ways to beat a case of the blahs is to change your appearance in some way. It doesn't have to be a major head-to-toe makeover. The smallest change can elevate your mood. This is an especially effective technique to use if the blahs you are feeling are in any way connected to how you look at the moment.

Get a haircut. Notice that I didn't say get a trim. A trim will not do. Grab a couple of hair magazines and look for a new hairstyle. You will be amazed at how different you feel when you get a haircut. It doesn't have to be drastically different. It could be the addition of bangs, or adding a few highlights. No matter how big or small the change, you will feel instantly different when you look in the mirror afterwards.

Give yourself a manicure. This is for guys too by the way. The word 'man' is in the word manicure after all! Obviously I am not suggesting you guys get polish put on your nails, but trimming and filing your nails is a good practice. The best dressed men always have their hands well groomed.

A manicure or pedicure is a small form of pampering that many people just don't take the time to do. This little change in your appearance can have a big effect on how you feel about yourself. When you take time to focus on yourself like this you send a powerful message to your subconscious. It says "I care about you!" because you are caring enough to do something nice for yourself.

Get some new makeup ladies. If you have been using the same eye shadow for as long as you can remember, it is time for an updated look. Go visit the cosmetics counter and get some advice on how to change your look to suit the person you are now. Maybe try out some new colour. Remember how much colour can effect you? What you put on your face can be a great pick-me-up.

Get some new clothes. The term dress for success is used for a reason. If you dress in age-appropriate attire people will take you more seriously. You will attract the right kind of mate. Your boss will take you more seriously. You will feel more confident and sexy.

You don't need to get brand new clothes by the way. If you are on a tight budget, check out the local thrift store. I have found some really cool items at these stores. Lots of the clothes there are in great condition. You can find designer duds at a fraction of the cost. Who cares if they are 'last season'? You'll look hot and that's all that matters when you are thinking about raising your positivity.

Live Events

The purpose of life is to live it, to taste experience to the utmost, to reach out eagerly and without fear for newer and richer experience.

– Eleanor Roosevelt

Instead of going to a bunch of movies during the year, I like to save up my money and go to a few live events. There is nothing quite like seeing people perform on stage. To watch these live shows and events is a real treat.

Going to the theatre is wonderful. Watching the actors onstage, knowing that at any moment they could totally mess up a line. I find myself reveling in their art. I love the entire show. The orchestra accentuating the acting; the backdrops and the makeup; the whole experience is other-worldly. Live theatre brings the land of make-believe alive before your eyes.

Concerts are always a blast to go to. Live music is so much more earthy and primal than music on the radio. You get to watch the music being created. You get to see the drummer banging away at the drums; the guitarist and bassist strumming their notes, weaving them into the song. The way they move as they play, the energy they put into their music, is so inspiring to watch. I used to manage a local rock band and I never tired of watching them perform.

Live dance is something special to me. I used to go to the ballet every year with my Grandma Carson. I was enchanted by the way those dancers moved. They looked light as air. They were so graceful. Recently I became fascinated again by dance when I tuned into a reality TV show full of young dancers competing for money and recognition. I couldn't wait to see the next week's episode. There were so many styles of dance I had never seen before. I discovered ballroom, hip hop, and contemporary. All of it is so beautiful. I definitely intend to spend time watching live dance in the future.

Magic shows are fun to go to. Watching an illusionist is pretty cool. I have been to a big show in Vancouver. I left there feeling completely boggled by what I had seen. My mind couldn't wrap my head around it. I was amazed (and I'll admit a bit freaked out) by the tricks that guy pulled. Since that first show I have actually met a friend who is a magician. He is so good! I get to see him perform every Christmas Eve. He repeats some of the tricks but I love them every time. I have yet to figure out how he does any of the illusions. I hope I never do. The secrecy of magic is what makes it so fun to watch. It's fun to be spellbound.

Sometimes our souls need a little nourishment. We tend to get into a routine that lacks this. From time to time, do something that lets you feel deeply comforted. Some of these things are fun, some are relaxing, and some are challenging. All of these things are good for the deepest part of you; the part I call the soul.

So curiosity, I think, is a really important aspect of staying young or youthful.

-Goldie Hawn

Chapter 11

Eternal Youth

There are some things that really tap into your inner child. They bring back fond memories and take you back to a simpler time. People tend to become jaded as they get older. They lose their naivety and their sense of wonder. It becomes harder and harder to bring on a feeling of awe.

As a child you were probably full of curiosity and a desire to explore the world around you. Life was full of possibility then. You weren't hindered by the adult world. You were free to dream and to imagine what your life could be like.

Being an adult can be a struggle. Life gets busy. It becomes a combination of stress, obligations, bills, disappointments, heartaches and the like. If we let it, life can become a dismal place. We can lose ourselves to it. This doesn't have to be your reality. You can choose to live your life with enthusiasm.

Embrace Your Inner Child

When I was a child I had a vivid imagination. I created the most elaborate games and adventures in my own backyard. I would make-believe I was a witch brewing up potions, or a fairy flying around the bushes and trees. Some days I was Snow White talking to the animals. Other days I was a princess. I was full of an endless supply of ideas to act out.

When I reached my teens I became a scared and angry girl. I lost all of my imagination and curiosity. I squelched my dreams. Instead I focused my energy on secret crushes, being cool, awkward high school dances and smoking pot. It was a bizarre time of transition for me. It took a while to come to terms with no longer being a kid.

After I graduated high school, I started to remember the way I used to look at the world. I began to notice beautiful details again. There was less drama in my life. It was around this time that I started to renew my inner child. I would lie on the grass at a park and look at the clouds. I liked finding shapes and faces in them. I stopped avoiding puddles and would occasionally jump in them when I thought no one was looking. This may sound immature or odd but it made me feel alive and happy.

Sometimes we need to be silly. It's not smart to always take life seriously. When you let yourself goof off a bit it releases stress. If you don't want anyone else to know you are doing childish things then do them when you are alone. Blow bubbles in your house. I do it all the time now (under the guise of playing with my cats). Why do you think bubble-blowing is such a popular wedding activity these days? It's fun!

Sometimes when I just feel like letting loose, I jump in a big pile of leaves. I revisit little science experiments I did as a kid. I pull out art and craft projects I used to do like origami and paper maché. The simplest activities can make you feel young again. Why not find a Light Bright on eBay? Use it as decoration at Christmas. Find some retro games like Merlin and Concentration. Recapture the things you kind of miss from when you were a kid.

Light

In Vancouver, BC there used to be the coolest thing: the Laser Show. The Planetarium used to hold laser light shows. Laser lights were choreographed to music. I saw Beastie Boys, U2 and Pink Floyd versions. They would pump water vapour into the air and then flash these beams of coloured lights above your heads. The music would play loud and the experience would immerse you in this cool kind of trance. I loved it. They don't have the laser show anymore and I was so sad to see it go.

Light is an interesting thing. I've been curious about it for a long time. I remember the first time I saw a prism. I was intrigued by how a bent rainbow appeared when the sun hit it. I loved how crystals cast rainbows on walls. What a pretty sight.

There are great ways to incorporate light into your life. Some are more fun than others. Take fireworks for instance. I absolutely love fireworks! Big explosions of colour light up the sky. They linger in the air and then seem to drip back towards the earth. I have always felt amazed watching them.

Sparklers are another fun way to appreciate light. You get to hold a mini-firework in your hand. Spell your name in the air with it. Draw circles before it burns out. I brought sparklers to a New Year's get together this year. No matter how old you are they are always a hit.

I have already mentioned how great candles are. Think of all the places and ways you can use them. Fill a room with them to create a romantic mood. Make shadow puppets in their light. Be a kid again and blow them out on a cake.

Lastly there are campfires. This is light at its best in my opinion. I love staring into the fire and watching the hot flames lick at the air. It looks so hungry. I find myself mesmerized as I watch the flames attack the wood. Grab some friends and roast some marshmallows!

Fun Outings

Some of the easiest ways to recapture your youth are found at events around town. When was the last time you went to a circus? They are coming back into style you know. The advent of Cirque de Soleil started a renewed fascination with the circus. People all over the world gather to be wowed by trapeze artists. They get a riot out of the clowns. The circus I am thankful to say is back.

Carnivals are great escapes too. They hold simple pleasures like cotton candy and those little donuts. They also have rides. I don't know about you but I really love rides. I can't go on as many as I did when I was a kid but get me near a roller coaster and I must ride it. Bumper cars are a blast too. There is nothing quite like a carnival.

Aquariums are underwater adventures in the making. Go check out the regal Orcas. Playful Beluga Whales wait to squirt water at you. Dolphins put on a pretty cool show, as do otters. There are all kinds of neat creatures to look at and sometimes touch. I always liked looking at the turtles. My favourite sea creature is the Octopus. I think it is so weird how they change colour when they are scared or angry. They are like underwater chameleons.

Zoos are amazing places to recapture a childlike sense of wonder. I never had the chance to go to one as a child. As an adult I have been to two. I adored every minute of it. I love how big the elephants are and how tall the giraffes are. The low rumbling groan of the lions sent shivers down my spine. The zoo totally renewed my ability to feel awe.

Not all fun outings happen in the confines of a fence or building. Possibly the coolest times I have spent have been gazing up at the stars during a meteor shower. It makes me feel so small. I just stare up at the night sky and am filled with wonder at the vastness of it. Add to that the appearance of a shooting star or a satellite travelling across the heavens and my night is made. Once in a while you even get blessed with the Northern Lights or Aurora Borealis. That is a treasure that will bring out your inner child like none other.

Crying

Crying is cleansing. There's a reason for tears, happiness or sadness.

—Dionne Warwick

This one may come as a surprise but think back to when you were a kid. Remember how a good hard cry would wear you out. This can be a great way to get the negativity out of you to make room for feeling good.

The other day I was feeling a bit down. I couldn't really pinpoint why, I was just kind of feeling lonely. I had been spending enough time with friends and family so I was confused by the feeling of loneliness. Then it hit me. I was spending a holiday weekend alone again. I have been single for quite a while and I just started to feel frustrated and fed up about that. I realized I'm tired of being the only on in my family that isn't paired up; the single one at parties.

I found myself tearing up a bit so I just let it loose. I wallowed in it for a while. Not long; maybe 15 minutes. I cried and I muttered to myself about what was on my mind. My fears and my frustrations came to the forefront and I just let them all out. Crying can be very therapeutic. Tears actually release stress chemicals from the body, so if you feel the need to cry, do it. Don't bottle it up. Don't squelch it. Let the tears run down your face and allow them to provide the healing they are so good at giving.

After my good hard cry I felt so much better. I hadn't denied myself the need to grieve a situation I don't know how long I'll be in. I faced it and was honest with myself. Kids do this all the time. Why stop doing it when you are an adult when it is so obviously helpful? This is your party, so cry if you want to. Just make sure to find a way to shift your energy when you are done. I put on a comedy TV show and ended my night feeling perfectly at peace.

Being an adult is a part of life. There is really no avoiding it. Responsibilities will catch up with you eventually. Thankfully you don't have to let your sense of wonder and curiosity die as a result. If you take the time to embrace your inner child you will always have access to imagination and dreams. I encourage you to let loose once in a while. This will keep you eternally youthful. Be the adult the kid in you would want you to be.

Epilogue

There is no right or wrong way to be happy. However you get there is perfect for you. Increasing positivity is a very personal journey. Sometimes you will struggle with it. Other times it will be as easy as breathing. Be patient with yourself. It isn't a race. This is your life. Choose every day, to make it the best life you can.

Choose to be happy and you will be. Make it a daily practice. Let it become part of your routine; part of who you are. With every hurdle you overcome, you will be stronger and wiser.

Embrace the parts of yourself that are secret and let them shine. Look at yourself the way your loved ones see you. See that you are more than just the sum of your parts. You are special. You are unique.

My sincere hope is that at least one thing in this book helps you find happiness. I thank you for trusting me with your time. It has been a real pleasure sharing my thoughts with you.

Appendix

Websites Worth Checking Out:

For Fun:
meetup.com - a great place to meet friends

pinterest.com - to find out what you like

stumbleupon.com - explore new things

thesmashbook.com - art journaling techniques

Therapies:
tcmcanada.org - Acupuncture info

acupuncture.com

reiki.ca – Canadian Reiki Association

christianreiki.org

iarp.org – International Association of Reiki
Practitioners

chiropracticcanada.ca – Canadian Chiropractic
Association

acatoday.org – American Chiropractic Association

catainfo.ca – Canadian Art Therapy Association

arttherapy.org – American Art Therapy Association

canadianhypnotherapyassociation.ca

hypnosis.edu/aha – American Hypnosis Association

Miscellaneous Sites:

doyogawithme.com – site with free yoga videos

vitalaffirmations.com – free affirmations to use

masaru-emoto.net – Dr. Emoto's website on his
water crystals study

Recommended Reading:

The Secret – Rhonda Byrne

The Power – Rhonda Byrne

The Power of Positive Thinking – Norman Vincent
Peale

I Can Make You Happy – Paul McKenna

Feel the Fear and Do It Anyway – Susan Jeffers

You Can Heal Your Life – Louise L. Hay

The Five Love Languages – Gary Chapman

Hypnosis Secrets of the Mind – Michael Streeter

The Power of Stillness – Tobin Blake

Classical Music Suggestions

Look up the following composers online or in music
stores. These are famous artists and will serve as a
good introduction to classical music as some of their
music will already be familiar. Once you get used to
the kinds of styles that you prefer, you can use

websites such as Pandora.com and Amazon.com to find other composers.

Bach

Vivaldi

Brahms

Beethoven

Chopin

Mozart

Handel

Telemann

Schumann

Boccherini

Debussy

Tchaikovsky

19689826R00110

Made in the USA
Charleston, SC
07 June 2013